Map Key

Other Titles of Interest

60 Hikes within 60 Miles: Los Angeles, by Laura Randall

Visit www.menasharidge.com for the full skinny on all the latest Menasha Ridge Press how-to and where-to outdoor guidebooks

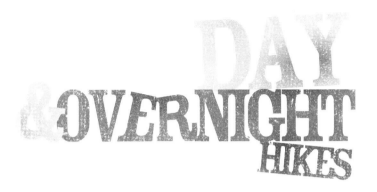

Palm Springs

Laura Randall

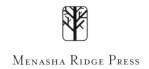

Menasha Ridge Press

DISCLAIMER

This book is meant only as a guide to select trails in the vicinity of the Palm Springs and does not guarantee hiker safety in any way—you hike at your own risk. Neither Menasha Ridge Press nor Laura Randall is liable for property loss or damage, personal injury, or death that result in any way from accessing or hiking the trails described in the following pages. Please be aware that hikers have been injured in the Palm Springs area. Be especially cautious when walking on or near boulders, steep inclines, and drop-offs, and do not attempt to explore terrain that may be beyond your abilities. To help ensure an uneventful hike, please read carefully the introduction to this book, and perhaps get further safety information and guidance from other sources. Familiarize yourself thoroughly with the areas you intend to visit before venturing out. Ask questions, and prepare for the unforeseen. Familiarize yourself with current weather reports, maps of the area you intend to visit, and any relevant park regulations.

Copyright © 2008 by Laura Randall
All rights reserved
Published by Menasha Ridge Press
Printed in the United States of America
Distributed by Publishers Group West
First edition, first printing

Text and cover design by Ian Szymkowiak (Palace Press International)
Cover photograph by Laura Randall
Author photograph by John Kimble
Cartography and elevation profiles by Laura Randall,
    Scott McGrew, and Lohnes+Wright

Library of Congress Cataloging-in-Publication Data
    Randall, Laura, 1967–
        Day & overnight hikes Palm Springs / Laura Randall. — 1st ed.
            p. cm.
        Includes index.
        ISBN-13: 978-0-89732-981-1
        ISBN-10: 0-89732-981-3
        1. Hiking—California—Palm Springs Region—Guidebooks.
            2. Palm Springs Region (Calif.)—Guidebooks. I. Title.
    GV199.42.C22R36 2008
    917.94'97—dc22
                                        2007038625

Menasha Ridge Press
P.O. Box 43673
Birmingham, Alabama 35243
www.menasharidge.com

Table of Contents

DAY HIKES

INDIAN CANYONS

PALM SPRINGS

OVERNIGHT HIKES

For John

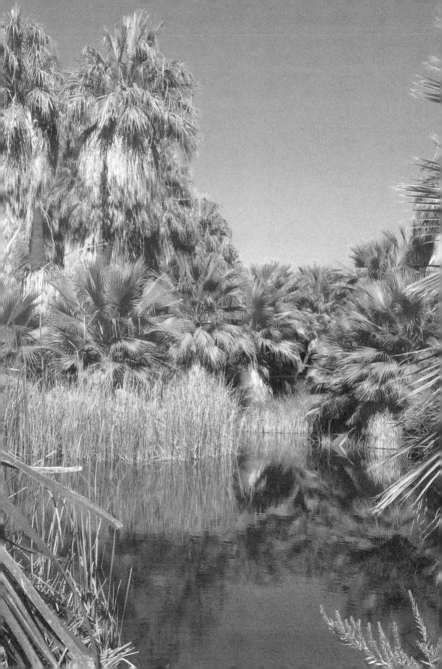

Acknowledgments

Thanks to the following folks for helping to make this book a reality: Jim Foote and the staff at the Palm Springs–South Coast field office of the Bureau of Land Management; the staff of the Idyllwild Ranger Station; Mary Perry of the Palm Springs Tourism Bureau; and everyone at Menasha Ridge Press. Thanks also to Julie Makinen, Mark Magers, and Linda Yoshino for hitting the trails with me, and to the Coachella Valley and Desert Trails Hiking clubs for organizing regular hikes in the Palm Springs area and welcoming anyone who wants to join them. Most of all, thanks to John Kimble, who introduced me to Palm Springs years ago and whose fondness for the Southern California desert helped spark my own enthusiasm for the area.

Preface

Palm Springs often brings to mind images of palm-lined golf courses and swimming pools surrounded by lounge chairs, not rugged hiking trails for all levels of fitness and age. Yet the striking mountain ranges that frame this desert resort are full of winding trails that lead to natural palm groves, year-round waterfalls and streams, and cactus-spiked desert terrain. It may be near two other great natural spaces—Joshua Tree National Park and Anza-Borrego Desert State Park, but the Palm Springs area is a hiking destination in its own right. The Indian Canyons, where the Agua Caliente tribe of Cahuilla Indians once spent their summers, have dozens of trails, from easy half-mile jaunts to arduous treks that link to the 2,650-mile Pacific Crest Trail and Idyllwild on the other side of the San Jacinto Mountains. Four of the canyons—Palm, Andreas, Murray, and Fern—are clustered together at the south end of town, and another, Tahquitz, sits just off Palm Canyon Drive, Palm Springs's main drag.

To the north, the preserves of the Coachella Valley and Big Morongo Canyon are lovingly cared-for oases of palm groves, canyon washes, and tidal marshes that stand as a testament to the importance and dedication of volunteers. And in Palm Springs and neighboring towns like Palm Desert and Rancho Mirage, officials have worked with the Bureau of Land Management and others in recent years to improve and expand a network of trails, while at the same time keeping the area safe for the many forms of wildlife that inhabit it.

Desert trails come with their own unique sets of challenges. Hiking many of them during the summer months, when temperatures hit the triple digits, isn't a rational option for novice hikers. Parts of the Santa Rosa and San Jacinto mountains are prime habitat for the endangered peninsular bighorn sheep, and many trails are closed to dogs year-round because encounters with them tend to drive the sheep away. Other areas, like Clara Burgess and Boo Hoff in La Quinta, are closed to all hikers during lambing season from January to June. I've noted this for individual trails, but it's always good to check with the Bureau of Land Management or local recreation departments before hiking in or near a sensitive habitat area.

None of the trails in Palm Springs and the other desert cities described in this book allow overnight camping, but I include several hikes in the nearby Santa Rosa and San Jacinto mountains with good camping options. Idyllwild, a small mountain town with four seasons and many charming inns and shops, is a scenic 40-mile drive away and may be used as a base for these hikes. Nearby, the dense forested mountains and cool, pine-scented air offer a nice balance to the stark brown hillsides and sandy washes that dominate many of the Palm Springs trails.

This book offers more than 30 hikes within less than an hour's drive of Palm Springs. Some of them, like San Jacinto Peak and the North and South Lykken trails, have been around for decades and have been described with adoration by everyone from John Muir to nature-loving bloggers. Other hikes in the book, like Hopalong Cassidy and the Desert Hot Springs trails, are either newly developed or out of the way—they offer new and different experiences for even longtime hikers in the area. Though all of the hikes in Idyllwild are listed as overnight hikes because they offer camping options, most of them can also be hiked in a day; just be sure to allow enough time to return to the trailheads by sunset. (See the individual hike entries for more details.)

Whatever the reason you've chosen to visit or live in the Palm Springs area, hiking its trails will give you a real appreciation for the area's natural history and the way things were long before

Frank Sinatra and the Hollywood Rat Pack showed up. From the herds of bighorn sheep that still roam the hillsides to the hidden palm oases that helped the Agua Caliente Indians survive the searing hot summers centuries ago, there's much more going on around this stark desert landscape than one could ever initially imagine.

—Laura Randall

Top Recommended Hikes

Best Overall Hikes

7   Clara Burgess Trail
12   South Lykken Trail
25   Cedar Springs Trail
30   San Jacinto Peak
31   South Ridge Trail

Most Scenic Hikes

25   Cedar Springs
30   San Jacinto Peak

Most Difficult Hikes

30   San Jacinto Peak
31   South Ridge Trail
32   Spitler Peak Trail

Easiest Hikes

1   Andreas Canyon Trail
28   Hurkey Creek Trail

Best Maintained Trails

4   Tahquitz Canyon Trail
14   Art Smith Trail
16   Bump and Grind Trail
30   San Jacinto Peak

Best for Solitude

13   Vargas Palms
18   Desert Hot Springs: Swiss Canyon Trail
25   Cedar Springs Trail
29   Ramona Trail

Best for Children

1   Andreas Canyon Trail
4   Tahquitz Canyon Trail
15   Big Morongo Canyon Trail
28   Herkey Creek Trail

Hikes with Dogs

10   North Lykken Trail
12   South Lykken Trail
23   Black Mountain Road Trail
28   Hurkey Creek Trail

Steep Hikes

6   Araby Trail
7   Clara Burgess Trail
9   Museum Trail
10   North Lykken Trail
30   San Jacinto Peak
31   South Ridge Trail
32   Spitler Peak Trail

Flat Hikes

1   Andreas Canyon Trail
4   Tahquitz Canyon Trail
13   Vargas Palms
28   Hurkey Creek Trail

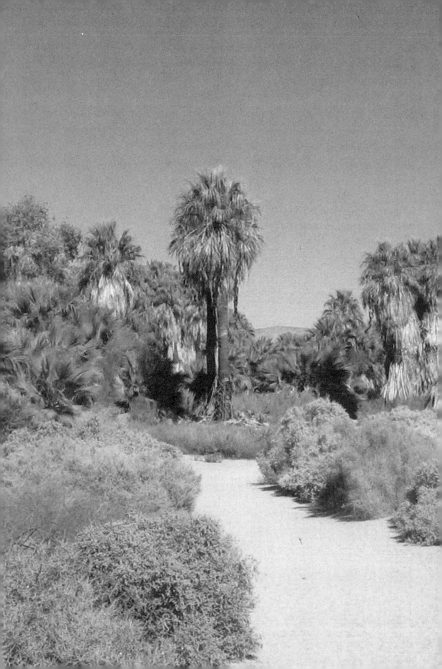

Introduction

How to Use This Guidebook

THE OVERVIEW MAP AND OVERVIEW MAP KEY

Use the overview map on the inside front cover to find the exact
locations of each hike's primary trailhead. Each hike's number
appears on the overview map, on the map key facing the overview
map, and in the table of contents. When flipping through the book,
a hike's full profile is easy to locate by watching for the hike number
at the top of each page.

The book is organized by region, as indicated in the table of
contents. The hikes within each region are noted as one-way day
hikes, loop day hikes, or overnight loop hikes (see page 167). A map
legend that details the symbols found on trail maps appears on the
inside back cover.

TRAIL MAPS

Each hike contains a detailed map that shows the trailhead, the route,
significant features, facilities, and topographic landmarks such as
creeks, overlooks, and peaks. The author gathered map data by
carrying a GPS unit Garmin Etrex Legend while hiking. This data
was downloaded into a digital mapping program Topo USA and pro-
cessed by expert cartographers to produce the highly accurate maps
found in this book. Each trailhead's GPS coordinates are included
with each profile.

ELEVATION PROFILES

Corresponding directly to the trail map, each hike contains a
detailed elevation profile. The elevation profile provides a quick look
at the trail from the side, enabling you to visualize how the trail rises

and falls. Key points along the way are labeled. Note the number of feet between each tick mark on the vertical axis (the height scale). To avoid making flat hikes look steep and steep hikes appear flat, height scales are used throughout the book to provide an accurate image of the hike's climbing difficulty.

GPS Trailhead Coordinates

To collect accurate map data, each trail was hiked with a handheld GPS unit (Garmin eTrex series). Data collected was then downloaded and plotted onto a digital USGS topo map. In addition to rendering a highly specific trail outline, this book also includes the GPS coordinates for each trailhead in two formats: latitude/longitude and UTM. Latitude/longitude coordinates tell you where you are by locating a point west (latitude) of the 0° meridian line that passes through Greenwich, England, and north or south of the 0° (longitude) line that belts Earth, a.k.a. the equator.

Topographic maps show latitude/longitude as well as UTM grid lines. Known as UTM coordinates, the numbers index a specific point using a grid method. The survey datum used to arrive at the coordinates in this book is WGS84 (versus NAD27 or WGS83). For readers who own a GPS unit, whether handheld or onboard a vehicle, the latitude/longitude or UTM coordinates provided on the first page of each hike may be entered into the GPS unit. Just make sure your GPS unit is set to navigate using WGS84 datum. Now you can navigate directly to the trailhead.

Most trailheads, which begin in parking areas, can be reached by car, but some hikes still require a short walk to reach the trailhead from a parking area. In those cases, a handheld unit is necessary to continue the GPS navigation process. That said, however, readers can easily access all trailheads in this book by using the directions given, the overview map, and the trail map, which shows at least one major road leading into the area. But for those who enjoy using the latest GPS technology to navigate, the necessary data has been provided.

A brief explanation of the UTM coordinates from Victor Trail (page 39) follows.

UTM Zone (WGS84)	11S
Easting	542753
Northing	3733212

The UTM zone number 11 refers to one of the 60 vertical zones of the Universal Transverse Mercator (UTM) projection. Each zone is 6 degrees wide. The UTM zone letter *S* refers to one of the 20 horizontal zones that span from 80 degrees south to 84 degrees North. The easting number 542753 indicates in meters how far east or west a point is from the central meridian of the zone. Increasing easting coordinates on a topo map or on your GPS screen indicate that you are moving east; decreasing easting coordinates indicate you are moving west. The northing number 3733212 references in meters how far you are from the equator. Above and below the equator, increasing northing coordinates indicate you are traveling north; decreasing northing coordinates indicate you are traveling south. To learn more about how to enhance your outdoor experiences with GPS technology, refer to *GPS Outdoors: A Practical Guide For Outdoor Enthusiasts* (Menasha Ridge Press).

THE HIKE PROFILE

In addition to maps, each hike contains a concise but informative narrative of the hike from beginning to end. This descriptive text is enhanced with at-a-glance ratings and information, GPS-based trail-head coordinates, and accurate driving directions that lead you from a major road to the parking area most convenient to the trailhead.

At the top of the section for each hike is a box that allows the hiker quick access to pertinent information: quality of scenery, condition of trail, appropriateness for children, difficulty of hike, quality of solitude expected, hike distance, approximate time of hike, and outstanding highlights of the trip. The first five categories are rated using a five-star system. Below is an example:

1 Andreas Canyon Trail

SCENERY: ☆ ☆ ☆ ☆
TRAIL CONDITION: ☆ ☆ ☆ ☆
CHILDREN: ☆ ☆ ☆ ☆ ☆
DIFFICULTY: ☆ ☆
SOLITUDE: ☆ ☆ ☆ ☆

DISTANCE: *1–3 miles*
HIKING TIME: *40 minutes–1 hour*
OUTSTANDING FEATURES: *California fan palms; caves, unusual rock formations, year-round stream.*

The four stars indicate the scenery is very picturesque. The two stars indicate it is a relatively easy hike (five stars for difficulty would be strenuous). The trail condition is fairly good (one star would mean the trail is likely to be muddy, rocky, overgrown, or otherwise compromised). The four stars for solitude mean you can expect to encounter only a few people on the trail (with one star you may well be elbowing your way up the trail). And the hike is doable for able-bodied children (a one-star rating would denote that only the most gung ho and physically fit children should go).

Distances given are absolute, but hiking times are estimated for an average hiking speed of 2 to 3 miles per hour, with time built in for pauses at overlooks and brief rests. Overnight-hiking times account for the effort of carrying a backpack.

Following each box is a brief italicized description of the hike. A more detailed account follows in which trail junctions, stream crossings, and trailside features are noted along with their distance from the trailhead. Flip through the book, read the descriptions, and choose a hike that appeals to you.

Weather

Sunshine, low humidity, and high temperatures are the main features of the weather in Palm Springs. The average annual rainfall is less than 10 inches. Winter days are mild, though strong winds can sometimes make hiking challenging, especially to the area west and north of town around San Gorgonio Pass. Temperatures start climbing in April and May and routinely exceed 100°F during the summer months. The risk of wildfires is also extremely high. Hiking during those times is not recommended. Layered clothing is a good idea when hiking between September and May. Temperatures can fluctuate on the trails as you weave in and out of canyons and the mountains cast late-afternoon shadows across the terrain.

Air quality tends to be good overall because the mountains surrounding the area serve as a barrier to the smog that plagues the Los Angeles basin.

The average-temperature chart below refers to temperatures in Palm Springs. As noted above, temperatures in Idyllwild and around the San Jacinto Mountains can vary considerably and dip well below those reflected in the chart.

AVERAGE TEMPERATURE BY MONTH					
	Jan	Feb	Mar	Apr	May	Jun
High	70°	75°	80°	88°	95°	104°
Low	44°	47°	51°	56°	63°	70°
	Jul	Aug	Sep	Oct	Nov	Dec
High	108°	107°	101°	91°	78°	70°
Low	76°	76°	71°	61°	50°	43°

In general, the desert recreational season begins in October, when temperatures begin heading back down to the double digits and the lows are at or above 60. By mid-November through February, tent camping becomes more challenging as temperatures begin dipping into the low 40s at night.

Water

How much is enough? Well, one simple physiological fact should convince you to err on the side of excess when deciding how much water to pack: a hiker working hard in 90-degree heat needs approximately 10 quarts of fluid per day. That's 2.5 gallons—12 large water bottles or 16 small ones. In other words, pack along one or two bottles even for short hikes.

Some hikers and backpackers hit the trail prepared to purify water found along the route. This method, while less dangerous than drinking it untreated, comes with risks. Purifiers with ceramic filters are the safest. Many hikers pack along the slightly distasteful tetraglycine-hydroperiodide tablets to purify water (sold under the names Potable Aqua, Coughlan's, and others).

Probably the most common waterborne "bug" that hikers face is *Giardia,* which may not hit until one to four weeks after ingestion. It will have you living in the bathroom, passing noxious rotten-egg gas, vomiting, and shivering with chills. Other parasites to worry about include *E. coli* and *Cryptosporidium,* both of which are harder to kill than *Giardia.*

For most people, the pleasures of hiking make carrying water a relatively minor price to pay to remain healthy. If you're tempted to drink "found water," do so only if you understand the risks involved. Better yet, hydrate prior to your hike, carry (and drink) six ounces of water for every mile you plan to hike, and rehydrate after the hike.

Clothing

There is a wide variety of clothing from which to choose. Basically, use common sense and be prepared for anything. If all you have are cotton clothes when a sudden wind or rainstorm comes along, you'll be miserable. It's a good idea to bring a light jacket or some type of synthetic apparel and wear a wide-brimmed sun-protection hat.

Desert trails can be slippery, rocky, and framed by cacti and other plants with sharp spikes; ankle-high hiking shoes and long pants offer better protection than tennis shoes and shorts. Sport sandals are more popular than ever, but these leave much of your foot exposed. An injured foot far from the trailhead can make for a miserable limp back to the car.

The Ten Essentials

One of the first rules of hiking is to be prepared for anything. The simplest way to be prepared is to carry the "Ten Essentials." In addition to carrying the items listed below, you need to know how to use them, especially the navigation items. Always consider worst-case scenarios like getting lost, hiking back in the dark, broken gear (for example, a broken hip strap on your pack or a water filter getting plugged), twisting an ankle, or a brutal thunderstorm. The items listed below don't cost a lot of money, don't take up much room in a pack, and don't weigh much, but they might just save your life.

WATER: durable bottles, and water treatment like iodine or a filter

MAP: preferably a topo map and a trail map with a route description

COMPASS: a high-quality compass

FIRST-AID KIT: a high-quality kit including first-aid instructions

KNIFE: a multitool device with pliers is best

LIGHT: flashlight or headlamp with extra bulbs and batteries

FIRE: windproof matches or lighter and fire starter

EXTRA FOOD: you should always have food in your pack when you've finished hiking

EXTRA CLOTHES: rain protection, warm layers, gloves, warm hat

SUN PROTECTION: sunglasses, lip balm, sunblock, sun hat

First-Aid Kit

A typical first-aid kit may contain more items than you might think
necessary. These are just the basics. Prepackaged kits in waterproof
bags (Atwater Carey and Adventure Medical make a variety of kits) are
available. Even though there are quite a few items listed here, they
pack down into a small space:

Ace bandages or Spenco joint wraps

Antibiotic ointment (Neosporin or the generic equivalent)

Aspirin, acetaminophen, or ibuprofen

Band-Aids

Benadryl or the generic equivalent diphenhydramine (in case of
allergic reactions)

Butterfly-closure bandages

Epinephrine in a prefilled syringe (for people known to have severe
allergic reactions to such things as bee stings)

Gauze (one roll)

Gauze compress pads (a half dozen 4 x 4-inch pads)

Hydrogen peroxide or iodine

Insect repellent

Matches or pocket lighter

Moleskin/Spenco "Second Skin"

Sunscreen

Whistle (it's more effective in signaling rescuers than your voice)

Hiking with Children

No one is too young for a hike in the outdoors, but take special care
in the desert with its cacti, rough terrain, and severe weather. Most of
the hikes in this book aren't suitable for children. Fit children over

the age of 10 may be able to handle flat, short trails, but the lack of shade, remote location, and unforgiving climate make hiking with toddlers and infants inappropriate. Use common sense to judge a child's capacity to hike a particular trail. A list of hikes suitable for children is provided on page XIII.

General Safety

The desert can be a barren, intimidating place, but to those who take the time to prepare and explore this vast wilderness, the area reveals its natural treasure. Potential dangerous situations can occur, but preparation and sound judgment usually result in safe forays, even in remote areas. Here are a few tips to make your trip safer and easier:

· ALWAYS CARRY FOOD AND WATER, whether you are planning to go overnight or not. Food will give you energy, help keep you warm, and sustain you in an emergency situation until help arrives. You never know if you will have a stream nearby when you become thirsty. Bring potable water or boil or filter all found water before drinking it.

· WEAR STURDY SHOES, along with a hat and plenty of sunscreen.

· NEVER HIKE ALONE. Take a buddy with you out on the trails.

· TELL SOMEONE where you're going and when you'll be back (be as specific as possible), and ask him or her to get help if you don't return in a reasonable amount of time.

· STAY ON DESIGNATED TRAILS. Most hikers who get lost do so because they leave the trail. Even on the most clearly marked trails, there is usually a point where you have to stop and consider which direction to head. If you become disoriented, don't panic. As soon as you think you may be lost, stop, assess your current direction, and then retrace your steps back to the point where you went awry. Using map, compass, this book, and keeping in mind what you have passed thus far, reorient yourself and trust your judgment on which way to continue. If you become absolutely unsure of how to continue, return to your vehicle the way you came in. Should you become completely lost and have no idea of how to return to the trailhead, remaining in place along the trail and waiting for help is most often the best option for adults and always the best option for children.

• **BE ESPECIALLY CAREFUL WHEN CROSSING STREAMS.** Whether you are fording the stream or crossing on a log, make every step count and bring a walking stick or trekking pole for assistance. If you have any doubt about maintaining your balance on a log, go ahead and ford the stream instead.

• **BE CAREFUL AT OVERLOOKS.** While these areas may provide spectacular views, they are potentially hazardous. Stay back from the edge and be absolutely sure of your footing; a misstep can mean a nasty and possibly fatal fall.

• **STANDING DEAD TREES** and storm-damaged living trees pose a real hazard to hikers and tent campers. These trees may have loose or broken limbs that could fall at any time. When choosing a spot to rest or a backcountry campsite, look up.

• **KNOW THE SYMPTOMS OF HEAT-RELATED EMERGENCIES** and prevent dehydration (drink water even before you are thirsty). There are three heat emergencies you should be aware of and know how to handle.

Heat cramps—painful cramps in the leg and abdomen, along with excessive sweating and feeling faint. Caused by the body's loss of too much salt, heat cramps must be handled by getting to a cool place and sipping water or an electrolyte solution.

Heat exhaustion—dizziness, headache, irregular pulse, disorientation, and nausea are all symptoms of heat exhaustion, which occurs as blood vessels dilate and attempt to move heat from the inner body to the skin. Get to a cool place and drink cool water. Get a friend to fan you, which can help cool you off more quickly.

Heatstroke—dilated pupils, dry, hot, flushed skin; a rapid pulse, high fever; and abnormal breathing are all symptoms of heatstroke, a life-threatening condition that can cause convulsions, unconsciousness, or even death. If you think a hiking partner is experiencing heatstroke, get him or her to a cool place and find help.

• **TAKE ALONG YOUR BRAIN.** A cool, calculating mind is the single most important piece of equipment you'll ever need on the trail. Think before you act. Watch your step. Plan ahead. Avoiding accidents before they happen is the best recipe for a rewarding and relaxing hike.

• ASK QUESTIONS. National Forest employees and park rangers are there to help. It's a lot easier to gain advice beforehand and avoid a mishap than trying to amend an error far away from civilization.

Animal and Plant Hazards

Ticks

Ticks are commonly found in brushy and wooded areas. Therefore, you are less likely to encounter them in desert areas than in other regions. Ticks, which are arthropods and not insects, need a host to feed on in order to reproduce. The ticks that light on you while hiking will be very small, sometimes so tiny that you won't be able to spot them. Primarily of two varieties, deer ticks and dog ticks, both need a few hours of actual attachment before they can transmit any disease they may harbor. Ticks may settle in shoes, socks, hats, and may take several hours to actually latch on. The best strategy is to visually check every half-hour or so while hiking, do a thorough check before you get in the car, and then, when you take a post-hike shower, do an even more thorough check of your entire body. Ticks that haven't attached are easily removed, but not easily killed. If you pick off a tick in the woods, just toss it aside. If you find one on your body at home, dispatch it and then send it down the toilet. For ticks that have embedded, removal with tweezers is best.

Snakes

Several types of rattlesnakes inhabit the Palm Springs region. I've never encountered one while hiking, but you should always be on the lookout for them. If you see one, give it plenty of room and leave it alone. When snakes have the opportunity, they escape from sight before you are upon them. Because snakes sense vibrations, a hiking

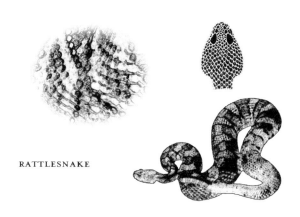

RATTLESNAKE

stick pounded along the ground as you walk gives them fair warning of your presence and allows them to slither off. When hiking in rocky areas, be careful where you step or put your hands. As with any wild animal, snakes are drawn to available water, so you may be more likely to encounter them near streams.

Mountain Lions

Mountain lions reside in the San Jacinto and Santa Rosa mountains, and have occasionally been spotted in the brushy foothills and riparian areas adjacent to them. Encounters are rare, but whenever you venture into an animal's habitat, the possibility exists. Here are a few guidelines for mountain lion encounters:

- **KEEP YOUR CHILDREN CLOSE TO YOU, OR HOLD YOUR CHILD.** Observed in captivity, mountain lions seem especially drawn to small children.

- **DO NOT APPROACH A MOUNTAIN LION.** Instead, give it room to get away.

- **TRY TO MAKE YOURSELF** look larger by raising your arms and opening your jacket if you're wearing one.

- DO NOT CROUCH OR KNEEL DOWN. These movements could make you look smaller and more like the lion's prey.

- TRY TO CONVINCE THE LION YOU ARE DANGEROUS— NOT ITS PREY. With as little movement as possible, gather nearby stones or branches and toss them at the animal. Slowly wave your arms above your head and speak in a firm voice.

- IF ALL FAILS AND YOU ARE ATTACKED, FIGHT BACK. Hikers have successfully fought off an attacking lion with rocks and sticks. Try to remain facing the animal, and fend off attempts to bite at your head or neck—a lion's typical aim.

Poison Oak

Although uncommon, poison oak does exist in the desert. Where water is present, you may find poison oak—recognized by its three-leaflet configuration—on either a vine or shrub. Urushiol, the oil in the sap of this plant, is responsible for the rash. Usually within 12 to 14 hours of exposure (but sometimes much later), raised lines and/or blisters will appear, accompanied by a terrible itch. Refrain from scratching because bacteria under fingernails can cause infection and you will spread the rash to other parts of your body. Wash and dry the rash thoroughly, applying a calamine lotion or other product to help dry the rash. If itching or blistering is severe, seek medical attention. Remember that oil-contaminated clothes, pets, or hiking gear can easily

COMMON POISONOUS PLANTS

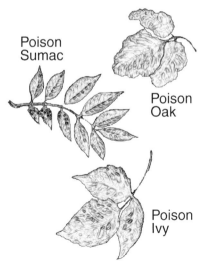

Poison Sumac

Poison Oak

Poison Ivy

cause an irritating rash on you or someone else, so wash not only any exposed parts of your body but also clothes, gear, and pets.

Peninsular Bighorn Sheep

Peninsular bighorn sheep inhabit dry, rocky, low-elevation desert slopes, canyons, and washes from the San Jacinto and Santa Rosa mountains near Palm Springs, California, south into Baja California, Mexico. Helicopter surveys conducted in the fall of 2004 indicated that approximately 700 Peninsular bighorn inhabit the United States. They have been listed under the California State Endangered Species Act (ESA) since 1971, but their population continues to decline. In late 2007, the Palm Springs-South Coast Field office of the Bureau of Land Management was developing a plan to help the hiking and bighorn sheep communities coexist peacefully, especially during sensitive times of the year like summer and lambing season. The plan isn't expected to radically change the trail system, but it will mean obtaining permits (which will be free and available at trailheads) for some trails near sheep habitat and more restrictions on bringing dogs on these trails.

The lambing season for bighorn sheep occurs between January 1 and September 30; during this time, hikers are required to remain on the trails and some trails, like Clara Burgess and Art Smith, prohibit dogs year-round for fear that they will drive the sheep from the area.

If you do spot a bighorn sheep in the area (but not on the trail), it's best to just continue walking at a steady pace along the trail. If the sheep is on or immediately adjacent to the trail (a rare thing), the hiker should stop and allow the sheep to move off the trail on its own accord, according to the Bureau of Land Management. The hiker shouldn't try to shoo or herd the sheep off the trail.

Tips for Enjoying Palm Springs and Idyllwild

Though most of these hikes are within easy reach of downtown Palm Springs and CA 111, it's easy to get lost or disoriented on the trails. Many of them quickly cut you off from civilization and disappear around mountain ridges and through thick desert vegetation. Know the trail and its surroundings before you go. Good maps are available at the visitors centers in Palm Springs and Palm Desert, as well as the Santa Rosa and San Jacinto Mountains National Monument on CA 74. Talk to the folks there before you go; most will be happy to brief you on what to expect in terms of trail condition, history, and wildlife.

In Idyllwild, stop by the Idyllwild Ranger Station before setting off, or call them at (909) 382-2922 before your arrival. The office has good trail maps, camping information, and knowledgeable staff. This is also the place to pick up wilderness and camping permits for trails like Devils Slide and San Jacinto Peak, as well as a National Forest Adventure Pass (see Backcountry Advice). Here are a few more tips for enjoying your time in the mountains and desert:

· TAKE YOUR TIME ALONG THE TRAILS. Pace yourself. The mountains and desert around Palm Springs are filled with wonders big and small. Don't rush past a jackrabbit or cluster of ocotillo trees to get to that final overlook. Stop and smell the wildflowers, if you're lucky enough to experience them after a rainy winter. Take time to revel in the cool shade of the towering palm groves you'll encounter on many of these trails.

· GET AN EARLY START ON THE LONGER HIKES, especially in winter, so you don't have to rush to make it back to the trailhead before dark. Late afternoon is a perfect time for shorter hikes as the air cools in winter and early spring and the sun casts dramatic shadows over the stark brown mountainsides. That said, take close notice of the elevation maps that accompany each hike. If you see many large altitude changes, allow for extra time. Inevitably, you'll finish some of the "hike times" long before or after what is suggested. Nevertheless, leave yourself plenty of time for those moments when you simply feel like stopping and taking it all in.

· DON'T WANDER TOO FAR OFF THE MAIN TRAIL unless you've done your homework. Many unmarked paths branch off from the main trails around Palm Springs: some eventually hook back up with the trail system; others dead-end at streams or sheer rock walls. If you're ever unsure, stick to the main trail (usually the one with the most footprints) and don't be afraid to ask other hikers for directions.

· WE CAN'T ALWAYS SCHEDULE OUR FREE TIME when we want, but try to hike the busier trails, such as those in the Indian Canyons and Idyllwild's Devils Slide Trail, during the week (though always with a companion). If you are hiking on a busy weekend, go early in the morning: this will enhance your chances of seeing wildlife and increase your chances of solitude. Use common sense if hiking the Palm Springs trails during the summer or early fall; get as early a start as possible and bring plenty of water and sunscreen. Avoid triple-digit temperature days altogether.

Backcountry Advice

A permit is not required to hike any trails within the Palm Springs area, and overnight camping isn't allowed on any of the trails in the desert cities. The San Jacinto and Santa Rosa mountains offer many campsites near the trails; many require a National Forest Adventure Pass, which costs $5 for a day pass or $30 for an annual pass. They are available at sporting goods stores and local ranger stations or by writing to the San Bernardino National Forest, 602 Tippecanoe Avenue, San Bernardino, CA 92408. A Golden Eagle pass, issued by the U.S. Forest Service, may be used in lieu of an Adventure Pass. Other day hikes around Idyllwild require that you pick up a free wilderness permit from the nearest ranger office before setting out. This is high-fire-hazard country; open fires are not allowed anywhere in the wilderness. Check with the U.S. Forest Service at (909) 382-2922 for other restrictions and updates.

Solid human waste must be buried in a hole at least three inches deep and at least 200 feet away from trails and water sources; a trowel is a basic piece of backpacking equipment.

Following the above guidelines will increase your chances for a pleasant, safe, and low-impact interaction between humans and nature. The suggestions are intended to enhance your experience.

Trail Etiquette

Whether you're on a city, county, state, or national park trail, always remember that great care and resources (from nature as well as from your tax dollars) have gone into creating these trails. Treat the trail, wildlife, and fellow hikers with respect.

· **HIKE ON OPEN TRAILS ONLY.** Respect trail and road closures (ask if not sure), avoid possible trespassing on private land, and obtain all permits and authorization as required. Also, leave gates as you found them or as marked.

· **LEAVE ONLY FOOTPRINTS.** Be sensitive to the ground beneath you. This also means staying on the existing trail and not blazing any new trails. Be sure to pack out what you pack in. No one likes to see the trash someone else has left behind.

· **NEVER SPOOK ANIMALS.** An unannounced approach, a sudden movement, or a loud noise startles most animals. A surprised animal can be dangerous to you, to others, and to themselves. Give them plenty of space.

· **PLAN AHEAD.** Know your equipment, your ability, and the area in which you are hiking—and prepare accordingly. Be self-sufficient at all times; carry necessary supplies for changes in weather or other conditions. A well-executed trip is a satisfaction to you and to others.

· **BE COURTEOUS TO OTHER HIKERS,** bikers, equestrians, and others you encounter on the trails.

Day Hikes
INDIAN CANYONS

1

The striking mountain ranges that frame this desert resort are full of winding trails that lead to natural palm groves year-round waterfalls and streams and cactus-spiked desert terrain

1 Andreas Canyon Trail

SCENERY: 🐾 🐾 🐾 🐾
TRAIL CONDITION: 🐾 🐾 🐾 🐾
CHILDREN: 🐾 🐾 🐾 🐾 🐾
DIFFICULTY: 🐾
SOLITUDE: 🐾 🐾

DISTANCE: *1–3 miles*
HIKING TIME: *40 minutes–1 hour*
OUTSTANDING FEATURES: *California fan palms; caves, unusual rock formations, year-round stream*

This short, scenic loop should be a part of any trip to the Indian Canyons. It's especially good for families, bird-watchers, and anyone who wants to experience the serenity of the canyons in a short period of time. The well-marked path leads past sheer rock walls and a year-round stream shaded by California fan palms to a seasonal waterfall and 1925 clubhouse once used by local hunters, then gives way to wide-open desert landscape. Though the best scenery can be found along the main 1-mile loop, the hike can be extended by 2 miles by picking up the easy horse trail on the north side of the road just before the parking-lot entrance.

🚶 The Indian Canyons, just south of downtown Palm Springs, are desert oases and the ancestral home of the Agua Caliente band of Cahuilla Indians. The area boasts year-round waterfalls, rocky canyon streams, and some of the largest collections of California fan palm oases in the world. More than a dozen trails of all levels snake through the canyons and connect to trails in Palm Springs and as far away as Idyllwild. Remnants of ancient life, such as irrigation ditches, stone shelters, and rock art, can be found along many of the trails. The entrance fees prohibit the area from being a regular hiking venue, but it's worth a visit at least once for anyone who wants to combine a hike with pristine desert landscapes and insights into an ancient culture. Detailed maps are posted at kiosks throughout the property and available at the entrance station and the Trading Post in Palm Canyon.

Look for the Andreas Canyon trailhead at the north end of the parking lot, just past a cluster of large rock formations. There is a

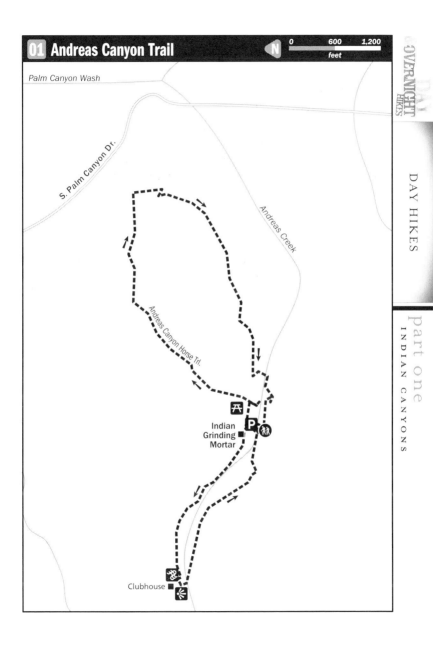

Palm Canyon Wash

S. Palm Canyon Dr.

Andreas Creek

Andreas Canyon Horse Trl.

Indian Grinding Mortar

P

Clubhouse

sign on the right just before the trailhead marked INDIAN GRINDING
MORTAR. The Cahuilla Indians used the bedrock mortars in front of
you to grind mesquite beans, acorns, and wild oats.

Follow the packed sand-and-rock trail down a gradual hill past
more rock formations. The stream, shaded by oaks, palms, and other
trees, is to your left. This is a great place for kids to splash around
and boulder-hop, especially in summer and fall, when water levels are
low. In the fall, the leaves on some of the trees turn bright yellow and
orange, making a nice contrast to the lush green palm trees.

The trail continues flat between the stream and towering rock
formations. At 0.25 miles, pass a signpost for Andreas Canyon
and take the path under a natural arch made of desert scrub brush.
Continue straight along the flat trail, with the stream to your left.
Soon the trail makes a brief ascent, then descends some natural rock
steps and comes within touching distance of more California fan
palms before hugging a sheer rock wall. Look for a small cave on the
right—the Cahuilla Indians once used this and other small caves in
the area for shelter. At 0.5 miles, the stream gives way to a pretty

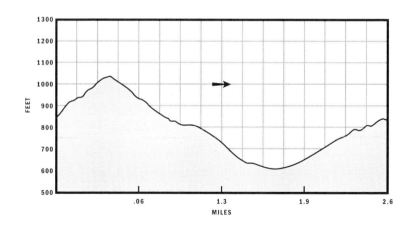

waterfall flanked by large boulders, another great place to stop and rest or have a picnic. I hiked this trail in the fall, when water levels were low, but the boulders can be slippery in late spring or after it rains. Be sure to wear sturdy shoes just in case.

To the west of the waterfall are two small stone buildings built on a hill; a chain-link fence bars public access. One of the buildings is the Andreas Canyon Clubhouse, the headquarters for a hunting club formed in 1923 on land once owned by the Southern Pacific Railroad. According to a sign, club members camped in the nearby streambed, using caches made of rocks. From here, the trail crosses a small wooden footbridge and loops back to the east; now the stream is to your left. Ascend a moderate flight of natural rock steps past distant views of rock formations and fields of creosote and desert sage. The trail levels for 0.25 miles before ending back at the parking lot.

Those who want to extend this hike can either hop on the Murray Canyon trail south of the parking lot, or pick up the Andreas Canyon horse trail to the east of the parking lot. This trail isn't as well marked as the main loop, but it's impossible to get lost, as the main road in and out of the canyon stays within sight the entire time. The hike is best done in the winter or early spring, since there is virtually no shade.

DIRECTIONS: From Interstate 10, take CA 111 south through downtown Palm Springs. Continue straight on South Palm Canyon Drive for about 3 miles to the Indian Canyons toll gate, where you can pick up a map and pay the entrance fee (at press time, it was $8 per adult, $4 for children ages 6–12). Turn right just after the entrance gate and go about a mile to the parking lot for Murray and Andreas canyons. Information: Indian Canyons, (714) 323-6018, www.indiancanyons.com.

GPS Trailhead Coordinates	I ANDREAS CANYON TRAIL
UTM zone (WGS 84):	11S
Easting:	0541785.5
Northing:	3735558.5
Latitude:	N33.809919°
Longitude:	W116.552504°

2 Maynard Mine Trail

SCENERY: ✿ ✿ ✿ ✿
TRAIL CONDITION: ✿ ✿ ✿
CHILDREN: ✿
DIFFICULTY: ✿ ✿ ✿ ✿
SOLITUDE: ✿ ✿ ✿

DISTANCE: *6 miles*
HIKING TIME: *4—5 hours*
OUTSTANDING FEATURES: *old tungsten mine,*
rock formations, desert vegetation, panoramic views

This out–and–back hike once served as the access route for a tungsten mine that operated during World War II. It begins in Murray Canyon and climbs steadily to the top of a ridge separating Murray and Andreas canyons for a total elevation gain of 2,100 feet, then drops over to a razorback ridge that leads to the mine. Explore the mine and a few pieces of rusty equipment left behind and enjoy the mountain and valley views before heading back. Sturdy hiking shoes and a hat and sunscreen are essential. Long pants are recommended because of the cacti and cat–claw acacia plants that line the path.

🚶 The Maynard Mine Trail is one of the more challenging trails within the Indian Canyons trail system. It starts on the south side of the Andreas and Murray canyon parking lot. Cross the small concrete bridge and look for a kiosk with a detailed map and a sign pointing you toward the Maynard Mine trailhead. Follow the path down a short hill to a row of horse-hitching posts, then make a sharp right and look for a large sign marked MAYNARD MINE. Follow the narrow loose-gravel path up the rock- and scrub-covered hillside. After a third of a mile of uphill walking, you will start to get nice views of the mountains and Palm Springs. Be careful of the cholla cactus and cat-claw acacia that can be found on either side of the path. Their short curved spines will cling to your clothes and can be very difficult to untangle.

At about 1.1 miles, the trail splits: head straight to stay on the main path. If you take the left path, you'll have to do some boulder

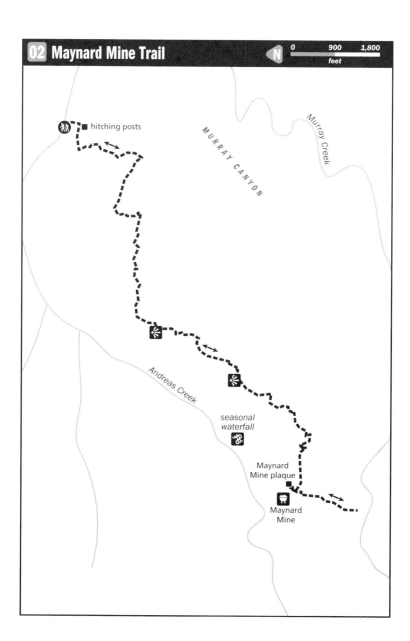

N

0   900   1,800
feet

hitching posts

MURRAY CANYON

Murray Creek

Andreas Creek

seasonal waterfall

Maynard Mine plaque

Maynard Mine

scrambling over steep terrain to get back to the main path, and it will slow you down a bit. At 1.4 miles, the trail reaches the mountain ridge and provides wide-open views of Andreas Canyon to the right. From here you can also see a long water pipeline snaking across the mountain ridge: this was once used by the Cahuilla Indians to deliver water into Andreas Canyon from mountain streams. To the far right are a few private homes perched on the mountain above the pipeline. Continue hiking south along a gradual incline up the ridge for another mile or so. If it's winter or early spring, look to the right across the canyon for a view of a gushing waterfall. At 2.4 miles, you will come to a signpost for Maynard Mine. You are at the hike's peak elevation of 2,800 feet, and it's all downhill from here.

The trail now follows a razorback ridge for another 0.4 miles to a clearing marked by a pile of mine tailings and a bronze plaque dedicated to Jim Maynard, the miner who first had the guts to lug a wheelbarrow and shovel to the middle of a barren hillside and start digging. The actual mine is about 200 yards north. Over the hill to the west are a few pieces of equipment used by miners, including an air compressor. Many visitors like to rest and have lunch here, since

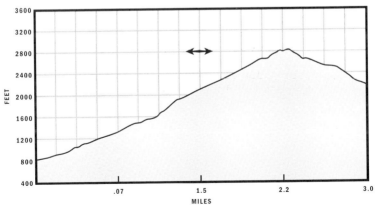

there are boulders for sitting and beautiful views of the mountains. To the southwest are Apache Peak, Antsell Rock, and Red Tahquitz Peak; the Pacific Crest Trail runs right below them.

In the fall, a small strip of deciduous trees that line the canyon are ablaze with red and orange. From the clearing, a steep dirt and gravel path leads down to a pretty canyon stream framed by these trees, but it's not recommended that hikers go beyond the mine. From the mine, you will have to retrace your steps back to the parking lot. The return is easier, more leisurely and graced by great views of Palm Springs and the large rock formations and palm oases of the Indian Canyons.

DIRECTIONS: From Interstate 10, take CA 111 south through downtown Palm Springs. Continue straight on South Palm Canyon Drive for about 3 miles to the Indian Canyons toll gate, where you can pick up a map and pay the entrance fee (at press time, it was $8 per adult, $4 for children ages 6–12), Turn right just after the entrance gate and go about a mile to the parking lot for Murray and Andreas canyons. Information: Indian Canyons, (714) 323-6018, www.indiancanyons.com.

GPS Trailhead Coordinates	2 MAYNARD MINE TRAIL
UTM zone (WGS 84):	11S
Easting:	3735725
Northing:	0541731
Latitude:	N33.760348°
Longitude:	W116.548575°

3 Murray Canyon Trail

SCENERY: ☘ ☘ ☘ ☘
TRAIL CONDITION: ☘ ☘ ☘
CHILDREN: ☘ ☘ ☘
DIFFICULTY: ☘ ☘
SOLITUDE: ☘ ☘ ☘

DISTANCE: *4 miles*
HIKING TIME: *2 hours*
OUTSTANDING FEATURES: *California fan palms; year-round stream with waterfalls, ancient rock formations.*

Wear sturdy hiking shoes for this moderate but mostly flat hike in the Indian Canyons south of downtown Palm Springs. After a brief dusty trek across sand and through desert scrub, the route weaves in and out of a stream lined with palms to reach a series of seasonal waterfalls known as Seven Sisters. Expect a moderate amount of rock scrambling and stream fording, especially in late winter and spring when the water levels are high. Keep an eye out for rattlesnakes during the warm summer months

🚶🚶 The Indian Canyons, just south of downtown Palm Springs, are desert oases and the ancestral home of the Agua Caliente band of Cahuilla Indians. The area boasts year-round waterfalls, rocky canyon streams, and some of the largest collections of California fan palm oases in the world. More than a dozen trails of all levels snake through the canyons and connect to trails in Palm Springs and as far away as Idyllwild. Remnants of ancient life, such as irrigation ditches, stone shelters, and rock art, can be found along many of the trails. The entrance fees prohibit the area from being a regular hiking venue, but it's worth a visit at least once for anyone who wants to combine a hike with pristine desert landscapes and insights into an ancient culture. Detailed maps are posted at kiosks throughout the property and available at the entrance station and the Trading Post in Palm Canyon.

From the parking lot, head east to a kiosk with a map and trail information. Turn left at the kiosk and follow the unpaved fire road past a small palm grove with a few picnic tables to another kiosk with

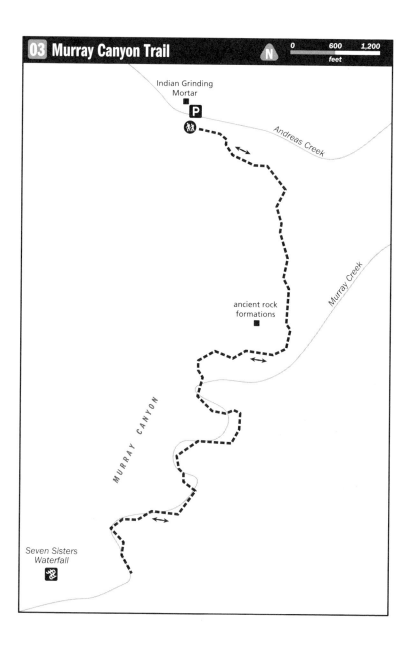

N

0   600   1,200
feet

Indian Grinding
Mortar

P

Andreas Creek

Murray Creek

ancient rock
formations

MURRAY CANYON

Seven Sisters
Waterfall

a sign for Murray Canyon/Seven Sisters. Take the sand-and-gravel trail straight beyond the kiosk as it begins a gradual descent into the canyon. After about 200 yards, the trail comes to a fork: go right, following the signs for Murray Canyon; to the left is a short path that leads to the West Fork Trail, a more strenuous hike that goes deep into the San Jacinto Mountains (there is another path that also hooks up with the West Fork Trail a little farther up Murray Canyon). The next quarter-mile is a flat walk past brown hillsides and desert vegetation such as creosote bush, cottonwood trees, and lavender. At 0.6 miles, the scenery improves as the trail wanders among ragged boulders; you can see the palm oasis in the distance and large rock formations to the right. Palm Springs and the Little San Bernardino Mountains are north, in the distance. At 0.75 miles the trail makes a brief descent into the palm oasis, and you'll reach the first of several stream crossings. This marks the beginning of Murray Canyon. Follow the signpost toward Seven Sisters to the right; the left fork (after the stream crossing) leads to the Coffman and West Fork trails.

The remaining mile is the toughest part of the hike, as the path weaves in and out of the palm oasis and across big rocks. To the left

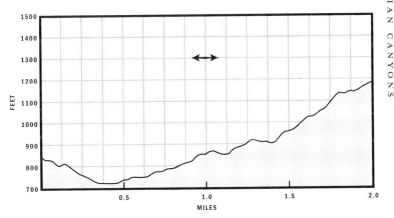

are stunning copper-colored rock formations, piled high and at wacky angles—a great photo opportunity. From here, the trail heads briefly into the shade of an arch of tall scrub brush, then continues east on a narrow, rocky course toward more palm trees.

At 1.2 miles, you'll come to another signpost for Seven Sisters. Beyond it, the trail continues its gradual ascent up a rocky hillside, with the palm oasis to the right, then heads down into the canyon. Now you are deep into the canyon, surrounded by California fan palms and natural pools—a world away from bustling Palm Springs. This trail gets a moderate amount of foot traffic, though, so don't be surprised to run into fellow hikers, and even the occasional equestrian.

At 1.7 miles, the trail crosses the stream again and heads uphill in short, easy switchbacks before dipping back down into the canyon. After a brief steep ascent of carved rock steps, the trail levels again. Be sure to stop here and look back for a fine bird's eye view of Murray Canyon. You've reached Seven Sisters, a series of waterfalls fed by natural pools and shaded by California fan palms. Don't count on all the waterfalls to be flowing, especially in the dry fall months. The best time to see them is April or May, according to canyon rangers. The area is dotted with big, flat rocks, perfect for having a picnic lunch by the water. You can also hike down to the pools and take a dip in the cool, refreshing water (test it first to make sure it's not too cold), or just make your way under the waterfalls for a unique view of the canyon.

From here, make your way back to the main trail and retrace your route to parking lot. There are also picnic tables near the parking area if you want to cap your hike with a lunch or snack before leaving the Indian Canyons.

DIRECTIONS: From Interstate 10, take CA 111 south through downtown Palm Springs. Continue straight on South Palm Canyon Drive for about 3 miles to the Indian Canyons toll gate, where you can pick up a map and pay the entrance fee (at press time, it was $8 per adult, $4 for children ages 6–12). Turn right just after the entrance gate and go about a mile to the parking lot for Murray and Andreas canyons. Information: Indian Canyons, (714) 323-6018, www.indiancanyons.com.

GPS Trailhead Coordinates	3 MURRAY CANYON TRAIL
UTM zone (WGS 84):	11S
Easting:	0541712
Northing:	3735677
Latitude:	N33.760777°
Longitude:	W116.548525°

4 Tahquitz Canyon Trail

SCENERY: 🐾 🐾 🐾 🐾	DISTANCE: *2 miles*
TRAIL CONDITION: 🐾 🐾 🐾 🐾	HIKING TIME: *1 hour, 15 minutes*
CHILDREN: 🐾 🐾 🐾 🐾	OUTSTANDING FEATURES: *waterfalls, rock*
DIFFICULTY: 🐾 🐾	*formations, Native American pictographs*
SOLITUDE: 🐾 🐾 🐾	

Framed by the San Jacinto mountains to the west, this figure–eight hike follows Tahquitz Creek on a gradual ascent past ancient rocks and plants to a stunning 60–foot–high waterfall. The $12.50 admission fee ($6 for kids age 12 and under) seems a bit steep when there are so many good hikes in the area, but keep in mind that it goes to a good cause: maintaining the canyon's current pristine condition after it suffered years of abuse. It's a particularly fine hike in the spring when the falls and creek are robust with water.

🚶🚶 Tahquitz Canyon belongs to the Agua Caliente band of Cahuilla Indians and is listed in the National Register of Historic Places. Tahquitz comes from the name of an Indian shaman who was banished to the canyon when he abused his powers. The tribe believes his spirit still lives within the canyon walls and that he is searching for the souls of those who get too close to his lair. Squatters lived in the area for decades before the tribe kicked them out and spent four years cleaning up the graffiti and vandalism that was left behind. The canyon reopened for guided tours in 2001; now it allows visitors to take self-guided hikes on a 2-mile loop trail (though guided hikes by tribal rangers are still held several times a day). You will be cautioned to stay on the trails during your visit.

The trailhead begins just behind the visitor center, where you pay the fee and receive a detailed map. Follow the rock-and-sand path southwest toward the mountains. An easy walk past creosote bush and barrel cactus gets you to your first sight: Sacred Rock, home of

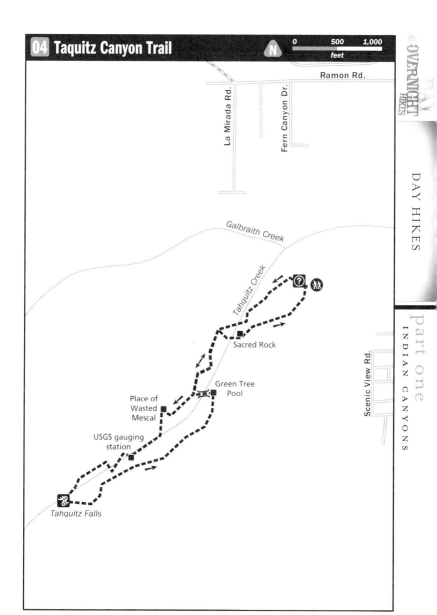

N

0   500   1,000
feet

Ramon Rd.

La Mirada Rd.

Fern Canyon Dr.

DAY OVERNIGHT HIKES

DAY HIKES

Galbraith Creek

Tahquitz Creek

Sacred Rock

Green Tree Pool

Place of Wasted Mescal

USGS gauging station

Tahquitz Falls

Scenic View Rd.

part one
INDIAN CANYONS

one of the oldest Cahuilla village sites. Stop and examine the painted prehistoric designs on the rock, then follow the path to the right, so you're on the right (west) side of the creek. Some of the other native plants to look for are desert apricot, white sage, Mormon tea, jojoba, and desert mistletoe.

At 0.6 miles, the path skirts a huge boulder, then reaches a fork. Stay to the right of the bridge (the left path also leads to Tahquitz Falls, but taking the westward route makes for a fun loop). Now the stream is to your left. Soon you'll come to a rusty gate and a water ditch on the right. This is known as the Place of Wasted Mescal and was used by the Cahuilla to bring drinking water from the canyon to the village. At about 0.8 miles, the trail skirts a long, thick water pipe on the right and moves closer to Tahquitz Creek, which was gushing impressively in late fall, even after a very dry summer. Follow the path up a series of natural rock steps. After passing a small waterfall on your left, you'll come to a U.S. Geological Survey gauging station, which was built in 1947 and is still monitored today. Continue heading southwest as the trail climbs toward the waterfall. At the 1-mile marker, the path hugs a

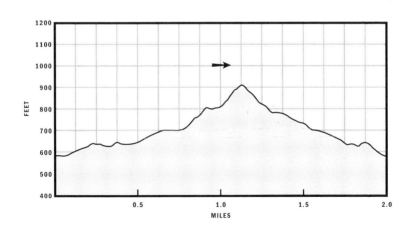

sheer granite wall on the right, then comes to Tahquitz Falls, a lovely 60-foot-high waterfall that seems to flow from nowhere high above you. Stop and rest here (even if you're not tired) and soak up the power of the place.

From here, the path loops around to the northeast and heads up, then down, a series of rocky steps. The creek is on your left. Soon you'll have great views of Palm Springs and the Gorgonio Mountains straight ahead. Contemplate the massive rocks that cover the landscape, and take time to appreciate their pristine condition. It wasn't too long ago that the whole area was littered with graffiti and trash. At 1.6 miles, you'll come to an overlook for Green Tree Pool, marked by a couple of large boulders: this is allegedly the site where a young Cahuilla woman was abducted and returned by Tahquitz himself.

Soon the trail curves left and crosses a small rock bridge. Just before reaching Sacred Rock again, you'll cross another small bridge, then meet up with the trail on which you started. Stay right to take the trail back to the visitor center (the path straight ahead is the way you already came). Piles of ancient dark-brown boulders line the hillside to your right, as more views of Palm Springs and the Coachella Valley come into focus. Soon the path begins another gradual descent on wide rocky steps, with the visitor center ahead.

Although I enjoyed the peace and solitude of hiking Tahquitz Canyon by myself, I can understand the appeal of taking a guided hike as well. I'm sure I missed some interesting stories and insights about the Cahuilla culture and the surrounding desert habitat.

DIRECTIONS: From Palm Springs, follow CA 111 to South Palm Canyon Drive. Make a right on West Mesquite Road and follow the signs to Tahquitz Canyon. The property is open daily from October through June, and on weekends from July to September. Information: (760) 416-7044, www.tahquitzcanyon.com.

GPS Trailhead Coordinates	4 TAHQUITZ CANYON TRAIL
UTM zone (WGS 84):	11S
Easting:	541321
Northing:	3741183
Latitude:	N33.809919°
Longitude:	W116.552504°

5 Victor Trail

SCENERY: ✿ ✿ ✿ ✿
TRAIL CONDITION: ✿ ✿ ✿
CHILDREN: ✿ ✿ ✿ ✿
DIFFICULTY: ✿ ✿
SOLITUDE: ✿ ✿

DISTANCE: *2.7 miles*
HIKING TIME: *1 hour, 15 minutes*
OUTSTANDING FEATURES: *California fan palms, desert and valley views, cactus scrub, seasonal stream*

This easy loop trail offers a nice introduction to the history and terrain of Palm Springs's Indian Canyons. The Victor Trail (via Palm Canyon) takes you under a sea of fan palms and past cactus scrub, a seasonal stream, and rock mortars that were used by the Agua Caliente band to grind fruits, seeds, and nuts 2,000 years ago. With its moderate 300-foot elevation gain and easy stream crossings, this hike is good for novice hikers or older children, though check in at the Trading Post about conditions before you go. There is no shade after the first mile, so a hat and sunscreen are essential.

🚶🚶 Begin this hike by descending to Palm Canyon via the concrete walkway just left of the Trading Post, a small shop and information center for the Indian Canyons. Once home to the Agua Caliente band of Cahuilla Indians, Palm Canyon contains the largest naturally occurring stand of California fan palms in the United States. The first mile of this trail is shaded by a thick sea of fan palms and winds past a stream that is lush and full in spring, but more of a trickle in late fall. Much of the path is a mix of sand and rock, so sturdy shoes are a good idea.

At 0.5 miles, you'll cross a small stream, which had been on your right. Continue 0.25 miles through the palm jungle, bearing left at a small wooden post marked PALM CANYON. Continue another quarter-mile to another signed wooden post marking a junction. Here the Palm Canyon Trail continues straight, but you turn left and uphill on the Victor Trail. You'll soon pass another trail junction

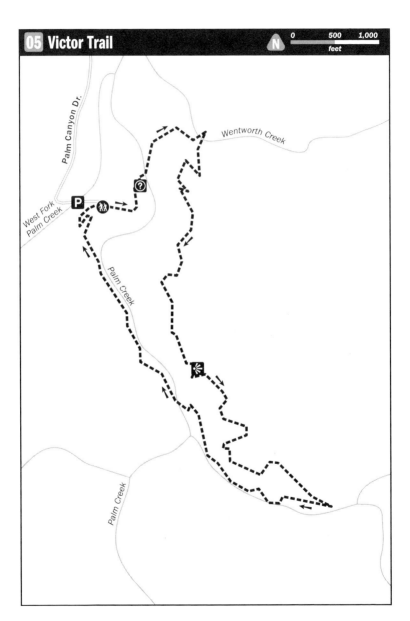

where the Vandeventer Trail joins on the right. Continue straight on the Victor Trail. As you climb the single, track, there are partial views of the San Jacinto Mountains to your left (west), and barren cactus-studded hills on the right. Soon you leave the palm trees behind (though they dip in and out of view for the rest of the way) as the path heads north around cactus-covered hillsides and ancient rock formations.

At mile 1.3, you'll come to another wooden post and a trail junction. Continue straight on the Victor Trail; to the right are the Fern Canyon and Hahn Buena Vista trails. At mile 1.4, the trail levels and reveals views of the Coachella Valley and the Santa Rosa Mountains to the north, then curves left and resumes its gradual climb. Enjoy more good views of Palm Canyon and the valley at mile 1.7, then follow the trail as it starts to swing right and uphill between huge, dark-brown rock formations. At 2.3 miles, you'll reach a four-way junction. The Fern Canyon Trail is right, and the Alexander Trail is straight. Stay on the Victor Trail by turning left, toward the Trading Post. From here, the trail dips back down into

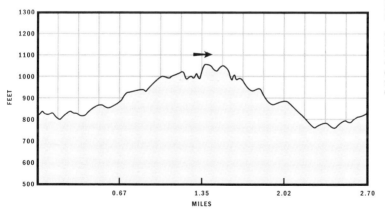

Palm Canyon. At 2.5 miles, head straight across a streambed (dry in late fall) and then follow the trail as it bends left. Soon the trail curves right and climbs past small rock clusters before reaching a kiosk with trail maps, a picnic table, and a small parking lot. Walk past the kiosk toward a fire-road gate, making a right before the gate and following the trail another quarter-mile back to the Trading Post parking lot. End the hike back at the Trading Post, which sells ice-cold drinks, as well as maps, postcards, and Native American art and jewelry. On weekends, the park offers ranger-led 1-mile hikes that include talks about the area's human and natural history.

DIRECTIONS: **From Interstate 10, take CA 111 south through downtown Palm Springs. Continue straight on South Palm Canyon Drive for about 3 miles to the Indian Canyons toll gate, where you can pick up a map and pay the entrance fee (at press time, it was $8 per adult, $4 for children ages 6–12), then continue another 2.5 miles to Palm Canyon and the Trading Post. Park in the lot outside the trading post. Information: Indian Canyons, (714) 323-6018, www.indiancanyons.com.**

GPS Trailhead Coordinates	5 VICTOR TRAIL
UTM zone (WGS 84):	11S
Easting:	542753
Northing:	3733212
Latitude:	N33.737841°
Longitude:	W116.537957°

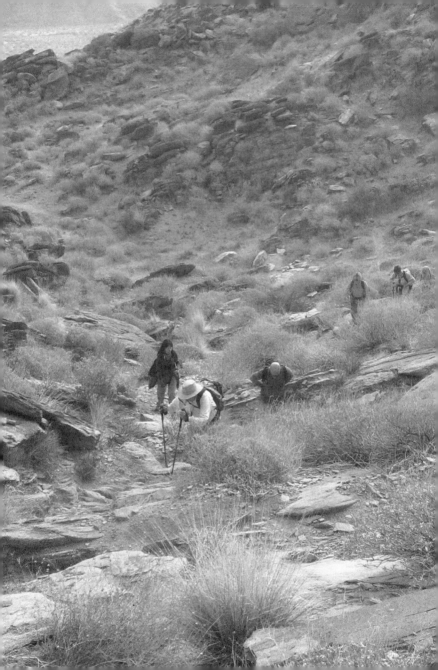

Day Hikes

PALM SPRINGS

2

The striking
mountain
range
that
frame
this desert
resort
are
full of
winding
trails
that lead
to natural
palm
groves,
year-round
waterfalls,
and streams,
and
cactus-spiked
desert

6 Araby Trail

SCENERY: 🌵 🌵 🌵	DISTANCE: *3 miles*
TRAIL CONDITION: 🌵 🌵 🌵	HIKING TIME: *1 hour, 30 minutes — 2 hours*
CHILDREN: 🌵	OUTSTANDING FEATURES: *desert and valley*
DIFFICULTY: 🌵 🌵 🌵	*views, cactus scrub, Bob Hope's former house*
SOLITUDE: 🌵 🌵 🌵	

This hike begins outside an exclusive gated community that was once home to Bob Hope and Steve McQueen, and turns into a strenuous ascent up shadeless switchbacks that comes within a stone's throw of Hope's former Jetsons-like home. Locals call it "the trail to Bob Hope's house," but it also serves to connect with other paths within the desert trail system, including the Garstin, Berns, and Clara Burgess trails. Boasting an elevation gain of 1,300 feet, this hike is appreciated more for its good cardio workout and celebrity connection than for its attractive views.

🏃 You can get to the trailhead from either side of the parking pullout. If you head west around the hillside, look for a small sign for the Araby Trail on the left, and follow it up the steep hillside about a quarter of a mile. This is a great cardio workout and leads to a lookout point over the surrounding community, but it gets a little confusing, and even intimidating, at the top. To continue on the Araby Trail, you will need to follow the trail east and walk around the left side of a foreboding chain-link fence with signs that warn you to keep away. It's a quick walk to the paved road, however. To the right is the gated community; you'll want to turn left and walk down the paved road until you see the trailhead on your right. It is marked by a small sign that says PALM SPRINGS TRAIL.

Those who want an easier route to the trailhead can walk up paved Southridge Drive from the east end of the parking lot, and look for the Palm Springs Trail sign on the left (east) side of the road.

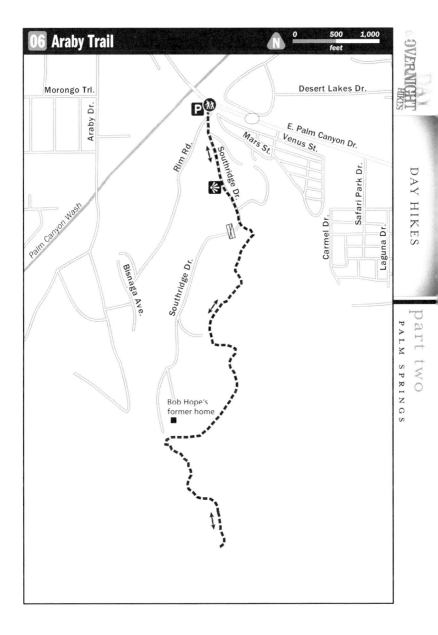

0   500   1,000
feet

N

Morongo Trl.

Araby Dr.

Desert Lakes Dr.

Rim Rd.

Southridge Dr.

Mars St.

Venus St.

E. Palm Canyon Dr.

Palm Canyon Wash

Bisnaga Ave.

Southridge Dr.

Carmel Dr.

Safari Park Dr.

Laguna Dr.

Bob Hope's
former home

The narrow gravel-and-dirt path starts a gradual ascent toward the south. To the left you'll see (and hear) traffic from CA 111; to the right is a view of the mansions that sit behind the big gates you just left behind. From here on, most of the scenery is desert scrub and brown hillsides. It is best hiked in the early morning or late afternoon, when the hillsides provide shade for parts of the trail.

At 0.6 miles, you'll pass more PRIVATE PROPERTY signs on the right, and the trail curves left. If you look up, you'll get your first glimpse of Bob Hope's house, but don't linger here too long. Better views await. The trail dips briefly before heading back up the mountain via wide switchbacks. At the 1-mile point, you will be within shouting distance of Bob Hope's house. The dome-shaped house is 25,000 square feet of glass and poured concrete and was designed by architect John Lautner. It has been called the "flying saucer house" and the "LAX terminal" because of its space-age appearance.

Continue past the house and its protective fence as the path meanders up the hillside. There is a paved street to the right that is part of the Southridge development, but heed the NO TRESPASSING

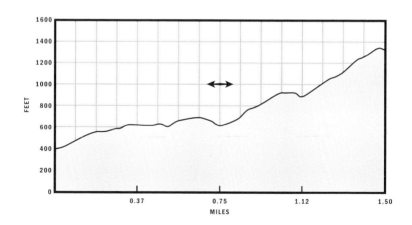

signs and continue hiking along the Araby Trail. Soon you'll pass a few big boulders that are among the rare resting places on this narrow trail. From here, you've got another half-mile ascent up wide switchbacks before you reach the mountain ridge. At 1.5 miles, you will come to an intersection and a sign for the Garstin and Berns trails, which form a single trail here that heads to the right. You can hook up with these trails, or turn around and retrace your route to Southridge Drive.

DIRECTIONS: From Palm Springs, follow CA 111 east toward Palm Desert. Make a right on Southridge Drive (if you pass Gene Autry Trail, you've gone too far east) and park at the turnout on the right-hand side of the road. Walk up the paved development road and look for the trailhead on the left-hand side; it begins about a quarter mile below a locked gate.

GPS Trailhead Coordinates	6 ARABY TRAIL
UTM zone (WGS 84):	11S
Easting:	0545305
Northing:	3739807
Latitude:	N33.797452°
Longitude:	W116.509726°

7 Clara Burgess Trail

SCENERY: ✿ ✿ ✿	DISTANCE: *7 miles*
TRAIL CONDITION: ✿ ✿ ✿	HIKING TIME: *3 hours, 30 minutes – 4 hours*
CHILDREN: ✿ ✿	OUTSTANDING FEATURES: *desert and valley*
DIFFICULTY: ✿ ✿ ✿ ✿	*views, solitude, cactus scrub*
SOLITUDE: ✿ ✿ ✿ ✿	

This hike within the Palm Springs trail system begins with a strenuous switchbacking climb, then levels for a mile or so of easy walking before returning to a final hardy climb to the top of Murray Hill. It requires you to take two other trails, the Garstin and Wild Horse, which eventually link to the Clara Burgess Trail. Ultimately, you arrive at a clearing with picnic tables and 360-degree views of the Coachella Valley. The path is well maintained and easy to navigate, with a total elevation gain of 1,500 feet. It's a good idea to wear sturdy shoes and bring a hiking companion with you. The last mile of this hike is closed from January to June each year because it is lambing season for the endangered Peninsular bighorn sheep.

👣 The trail begins at the end of Barona Road off Bogert Trail. Park on the street and look for the trailhead to the right of the road barrier that overlooks Palm Canyon Wash. The path, composed of packed dirt and small rocks, immediately climbs uphill via wide switchbacks. Soon you'll come to a signpost for Smoketree Mountain and the Shannon, Araby, and Wildhorse trails. Continue straight ahead toward these trails; you still have another 2 miles of robust hiking before you reach the Clara Burgess Trail.

The residential development you drove through to reach the trailhead is now below you on the right. Its landscaped yards and swimming pools are quite a contrast to the scrub-covered hillsides you're heading toward. After another hundred yards or so, you will reach another signpost; follow the Garstin Trail straight ahead. The Earl Henderson Trail branches left and continues on a flat,

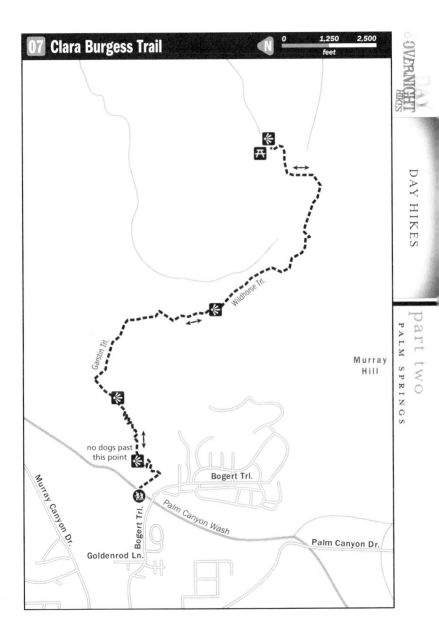

N

0   1,250   2,500
feet

Wildhorse Trl.

Garstin Trl.

Murray Hill

no dogs past
this point

Bogert Trl.

Murray Canyon Dr.

Bogert Trl.

Palm Canyon Wash

Goldenrod Ln.

Palm Canyon Dr.

northeast route to the edge of East Palm Canyon Drive. The Garstin Trail keeps its gradual ascent via wide switchbacks. At the half-mile marker, the trail skirts a small clearing with views of Palm Springs and a sign that says DOGS PROHIBITED BEYOND THIS POINT. This is a critical habitat for endangered Peninsular bighorn sheep, and wildlife experts fear that the presence of dogs may cause the sheep to flee the area.

From here, continue another half-mile to an unmarked fork; you want to follow the trail to the right and up the hill. Views of Palm Springs and the entire Coachella Valley come into view and weave in and out of sight the rest of the way up the mountain. After passing another rocky clearing, you will come to a signpost at 1.2 miles. Take the trail to the right toward the Garstin Trail. The trail to the left leads to Berns Trail, a connector trail that links with the Araby Trail. Now you'll really start to feel the solitude and total escape that characterizes this hike. I didn't see a single person when I hiked this trail on a Saturday afternoon in mid-November. It was a hot day, but the hillsides cast shadows on much of the trail, making it a pleasant late-afternoon excursion.

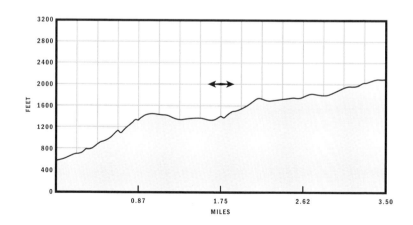

At 1.5 miles, the trail forks again; heed the wooden signpost that says TRAIL and continue straight on an eastern route. You will pass a large wood sign that says "Garstin Trail"; head straight, toward the sign for the Clara Burgess Trail.

At this point, the trail begins to climb again and turns to loose gravel for a bit, then goes back to packed dirt. You'll catch glimpses of the residential development again to your right, but it will seem like you're a world away.

At 2.2 miles, you will come to a clearing with a couple of big rocks overlooking the valley. This is a good place to stop and rest before continuing to Murray Hill; it's also a good turn-around point for those who prefer a shorter hike or those who despair of getting back to the trailhead before the sun sets.

To continue to the Clara Burgess Trail, head straight (east) along the mountain ridge. From here, the trail levels for an easy half-mile before reaching the Clara Burgess Trailhead and starting its final ascent to Murray Hill. At 3 miles, you'll come to a sign marking the Clara Burgess Trailhead. To the right is the Fern Canyon Trail, which leads south to the Indian Canyons. You want to continue straight and follow the Clara Burgess east over the hillside. Clara Burgess is a Palm Springs philanthropist. The views keep getting better and better as you walk. You're at an elevation of about 2,000-feet at this point, and you can see the entire Coachella Valley, as well as the little San Bernardino Mountains to the north.

At 3.4 miles, Murray Hill comes into view to the east. Another 0.2 miles of strenuous switchbacking brings you to the top. Once you arrive, you'll see why this hike is worth every drop of sweat. The panoramic mountain and valley views are breathtaking. Have some water and a snack at one of the two picnic tables at the top before heading back down the mountain. The hike back to Bogert Trail isn't likely to take as long, since the majority of it is downhill.

DIRECTIONS: From Interstate 10, take CA 111 south through downtown Palm Springs. Merge right onto South Palm Canyon Drive and continue to Bogert Trail, a paved residential street. Make a left and follow the street just past the bridge that crosses the wash. Make a left on Barona Road, the first road after the wash, and park at the end. The trailhead (unmarked) is to the right.

GPS Trailhead Coordinates	7 CLARA BURGESS TRAIL
UTM zone (WGS 84):	11S
Easting:	543521
Northing:	3737394
Latitude:	N33.776358°
Longitude:	W116.530468°

8 Earl Henderson Trail

SCENERY: 🐾 🐾 🐾 🐾	DISTANCE: *4 miles*
TRAIL CONDITION: 🐾 🐾 🐾	HIKING TIME: *2 hours*
CHILDREN: 🐾 🐾	OUTSTANDING FEATURES: *desert and valley*
DIFFICULTY: 🐾 🐾 🐾	*views, solitude, desert vegetation*
SOLITUDE: 🐾 🐾 🐾 🐾	

Named for local equestrian Earl Henderson, this unassuming horse and hiking trail begins in a typical desert–wash landscape, then zigzags around a mountainside to connect with other trails in the Palm Springs trail system. It's not the most dazzling of the Palm Springs trails, but it's a reliable, less strenuous alternative to the nearby Araby Trail. It has a moderate elevation gain of 400 feet and is popular with dog walkers and horseback riders from nearby Smoketree Ranch.

OPTION: The trail can also be accessed from Bogert Trail off South Palm Canyon Drive, at the same trailhead that leads to the Garstin and Clara Burgess trails. Follow South Palm Canyon Trail to Bogert Trail and turn left. After crossing a small bridge, turn left and park at the end of the street. Arrange for a friend to pick you up at Araby Drive, or retrace your route to Bogert Trail.

🏃🏃 From the parking pullout, walk across the street to the desert wash and begin hiking south amid the creosote bushes and tumbleweed. There is no marked trail for the first half-mile of this hike; just follow the sandy wash until you come to a trail junction for the Henderson, Berns, Garstin, Shannon, and Palm Springs trails (Note: Henderson refers to the Earl Henderson Trail, not Randall Henderson Trail, which is off CA-74 in Palm Desert.) Veer left on the Henderson Trail and cross a paved road to get to the actual trailhead. The other trails continue straight (south) toward a mountain. At 0.6 miles, you'll come to a large metal sign marking the entrance to the Earl Henderson Trail. Now you're on a single-track sand and

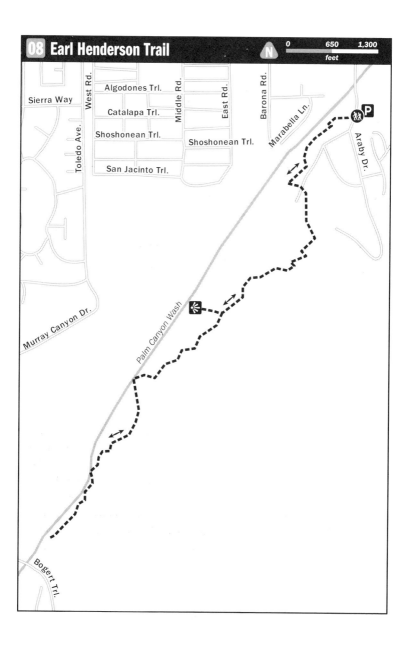

rock trail surrounded by brown hillsides and moving farther away from busy Palm Canyon Drive and its developments. After a short distance, the path begins to switchback up the mountain. The next quarter-mile is the steepest part of the hike.

At 0.85 miles, you'll come to a faded sign that says: 1968: THIS TRAIL MAINTAINED FOR YOUR RIDING AND HIKING PLEASURE IN MEMORY OF EARL HENDERSON AND LUCKY. From here, the path heads down a short hill, then levels and hugs the hillside for the rest of the way. Development creeps back into view in the distance to the right, but you will feel far removed from the homes and golf courses from up here. The canyon wash also comes back into view on the west. At about 1 mile, you will pass a small sign for the Palm Springs Trail, then pass a narrow trail on the right that heads west about a quarter-mile to a small lookout over the canyon wash and Palm Springs. Continue straight on the Earl Henderson Trail. At 1.75 miles, the trail heads downhill toward the canyon wash, then heads back up the mountain in a gradual ascent toward a trail junction that overlooks southern Palm Springs and the San Jacinto Mountains. From here, you have

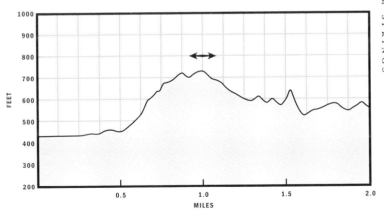

three options: Retrace your steps back to Araby Drive; continue your hike by taking the Garstin Trail southeast into the mountains; or take the path to the west down the hill toward Bogert Trail, and have someone pick you up there, making the hike 2 miles instead of 4.

DIRECTIONS: From Interstate 10, take the Palm Drive exit toward Desert Hot Springs/Palm Desert. Head south about 6 miles (Palm Drive turns into Gene Autry Trail) until you reach East Palm Canyon Drive. Turn right and go about 0.5 miles to Araby Drive. Make a left and go 0.45 miles to an unpaved parking pullout on the left.

GPS Trailhead Coordinates	8 EARL HENDERSON TRAIL
UTM zone (WGS 84):	11S
Easting:	0544902
Northing:	3739365
Latitude:	N33.793482°
Longitude:	W116.514096°

9 Museum Trail

SCENERY: 🐾 🐾 🐾 TRAIL CONDITION: 🐾 🐾 🐾 CHILDREN: 🐾 🐾 DIFFICULTY: 🐾 🐾 🐾 🐾 SOLITUDE: 🐾 🐾	DISTANCE: *2 miles* HIKING TIME: *1 hour* OUTSTANDING FEATURES: *steep rocky hillside, cactus and desert scrub, city and valley views*

This popular hike begins near downtown Palm Springs and crisscrosses the mountainside, gaining 1,000 feet in elevation in just 1 mile. It links with the North and South Lykken trails, as well as the very challenging Skyline Ridge Route (also known as the Cactus to Clouds Trail), a relentless, uphill climb to San Jacinto Peak.

🚶🚶 This hike is called the Museum Trail because it begins at the edge of the parking lot for the Palm Springs Art Museum, just off the town's main drag. Look for the sign that says WELCOME TO THE MUSEUM TRAIL at the north end of the lot. There's a good map of the trail system here. There is no shade along the trail; water and sunscreen are essential. Locals use this cardio-friendly trail as an outdoor gym, so expect to see a fair number of other hikers, especially on weekends.

The trail immediately begins to wind uphill, flanked by a rusty handrail on one side and piles of rocks on the other. Soon you'll reach a private road and gate to your left; cross the road and get back on the trail as it continues its ascent of the rocky hillside. Someone has painted big white arrows on the rocks that line the trail, ensuring that no one will get lost on the way up.

At about 0.75 miles, you will come to a clearing with views of Palm Springs and the distant mountains. From here, the trail heads west toward the rocky hills and away from civilization. It levels briefly, then makes its final brief ascent to a clearing with picnic tables and

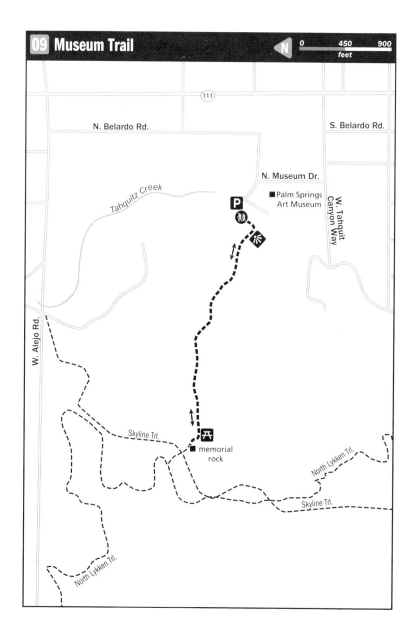

N

0   450   900
feet

(111)

N. Belardo Rd.

S. Belardo Rd.

Tahquitz Creek

N. Museum Dr.

P

Palm Springs
Art Museum

W. Tahquitz
Canyon Way

W. Alejo Rd.

Skyline Trl.

memorial
rock

North Lykken Trl.

Skyline Trl.

North Lykken Trl.

more fine views of the valley. This marks the end of the Museum Trail. It's a good place to rest before heading back down the mountain.

You can also access the North Lykken Trail from this point, though you hit it right in the middle. To pick up the South Lykken Trail, head north briefly before veering south, then follow a gradual descent down the hillside to the west end of Ramon Road. The North Lykken segment is shorter but more challenging uphill trek that ends near Chino Drive (see page 63 for more details on the Lykken trails).

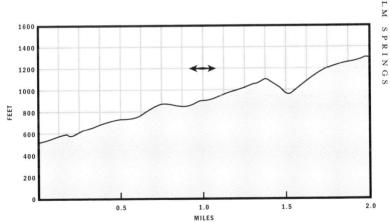

DIRECTIONS: From Interstate 10, take the CA 111 exit south toward Palm Springs. Continue on CA 111 as it turns into Palm Canyon Drive and passes through downtown Palm Springs. Turn right on Tahquitz Canyon Way, then make a right on Museum Drive. Park at the north end of the lot near the trail sign.

GPS Trailhead Coordinates	9 MUSEUM TRAIL
UTM zone (WGS 84):	11S
Easting:	541589
Northing:	3742862
Latitude:	N33.825476°
Longitude:	W116.549097°

SCENERY: ✿ ✿ ✿ ✿ TRAIL CONDITION: ✿ ✿ ✿ CHILDREN: ✿ DIFFICULTY: ✿ ✿ ✿ ✿ SOLITUDE: ✿ ✿	DISTANCE: *4 miles* HIKING TIME: *2 hours, 30 minutes – 3 hours,* *30 minutes* OUTSTANDING FEATURES: *desert vegetation,* *ancient rock formations, views of Palm Springs and the* *Coachella Valley*

The North Lykken Trail is the north half of the 9.5-mile Carl Lykken Trail, which weaves along a series of mountain ridges above downtown Palm Springs. This shuttle hike begins at the west end of Ramon Road in Palm Springs and ends at Cielo Road, off Vista Chino Road, north of downtown. It's more strenuous and less crowded than the south half of the Carl Lykken Trail (known widely as the South Lykken Trail) (see page 71), with a total elevation gain of about 800 feet, and it links with two popular trails—the Museum Trail and the Skyline Trail, also known as the Cactus to Clouds Trail.

OPTION: This can also be a moderate 3-mile out-and-back hike by turning around at the picnic-table overlook above the Palm Springs Art Museum, and heading back the way you came to Ramon Road.

🏃 Look for the trailhead on the right (north) side of Ramon Road and follow the narrow rock-and-sand path north as it switchbacks up the hillside for about 0.3 miles. You will pass a signpost where the trail levels and continues to curve north around the mountain ridge. The next 0.5 miles are a moderate walk along a mountain ridge accompanied by terrific views of Palm Springs and the Coachella Valley to the east. At 0.8 miles, the trail begins to climb again, then levels until it reaches a turnoff for the Museum Trail on the right. Continue straight to stay on the Lykken Trail, or take the Museum Trail 0.2 miles to a clearing with picnic tables. Here you can have a snack and enjoy the view before reconnecting

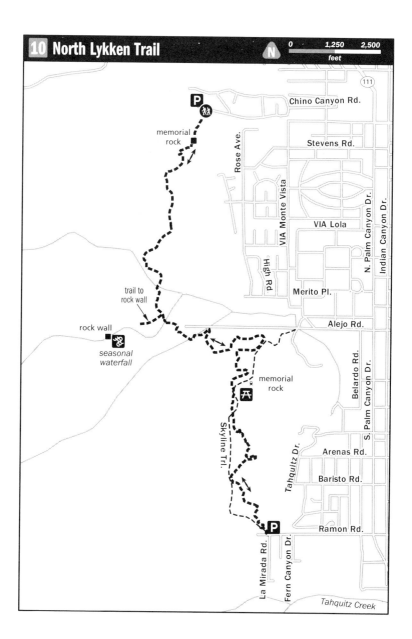

N

0   1,250   2,500

feet

111

Chino Canyon Rd.

memorial rock

Rose Ave.

Stevens Rd.

VIA Monte Vista

VIA Lola

High Rd.

N. Palm Canyon Dr.

Indian Canyon Dr.

Merito Pl.

trail to rock wall

rock wall

seasonal waterfall

Alejo Rd.

memorial rock

Belardo Rd.

S. Palm Canyon Dr.

Skyline Trl.

Tahquitz Dr.

Arenas Rd.

Baristo Rd.

Ramon Rd.

La Mirada Rd.

Fern Canyon Dr.

Tahquitz Creek

with the Lykken Trail. This is a good turnaround point for a 3-mile out-and-back hike.

To continue the shuttle hike, head northwest at the trail split and follow the Lykken Trail around the mountain as it begins a gradual descent into Chino Canyon. After walking about 1.3 miles from the trail split, you will come to an unsigned fork. Bear right; the left trail heads west for about 1 mile and dead-ends at a mountainside popular with rock climbers. Follow the trail across a canyon wash, then up a hillside to a clearing with picnic tables and another scenic viewpoint. From here, it's a short but very steep hike down the side of the hillside to Cielo Road. Wear sturdy hiking shoes and beware of loose gravel here. If you haven't left a second car or arranged for a pickup, turn back at the picnic tables and retrace your route to Ramon Road and the southern trailhead.

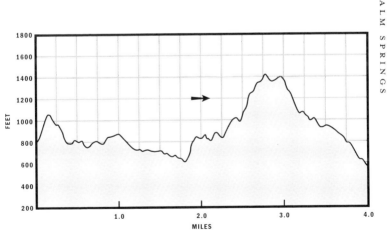

DIRECTIONS: From Interstate 10, take the CA 111 exit south toward Palm Springs. Continue on CA 111 as it turns into Palm Canyon Drive and passes through downtown Palm Springs. Turn right on Ramon Road and continue to the end. Park on the street.

To leave a car at the Cielo Road trailhead, turn left onto North Palm Canyon Drive from Ramon Road, and make a left on Vista Chino Road. Turn right on Via Norte, then left on Chino Canyon Road and continue through the residential neighborhood to Cielo Road. Turn left and look for the paved circular pullout on the left, just before the road ends.

GPS Trailhead Coordinates	10 NORTH LYKKEN TRAIL
UTM zone (WGS 84):	11S
Easting:	0541095
Northing:	3741820
Latitude:	N33.816063°
Longitude:	W116.554760°

11 Randall Henderson **Loop**

SCENERY: ♦ ♦ ♦	DISTANCE: *3 miles*
TRAIL CONDITION: ♦ ♦ ♦	HIKING TIME: *1– 2 hours*
CHILDREN: ♦ ♦ ♦	OUTSTANDING FEATURES: *ocotillo trees,*
DIFFICULTY: ♦ ♦	*cacti, and other desert vegetation, mountain views,*
SOLITUDE: ♦ ♦ ♦	*endangered Peninsular bighorn sheep habitat*

This loop hike near a visitor center is a good introduction to desert hiking, with a variety of plants and flowers, an easy–to–follow trail, and a moderate elevation gain of 400 feet. It skirts a major habitat for endangered Peninsular bighorn sheep: heed the warnings and stay on the marked trail. Dogs aren't allowed on the trail.

🏃 Begin this hike by walking the short quarter-mile nature loop trail behind the visitor center. Signs identify many of the desert plants and flowers you will see on the trail, such as sandpaper plants, brittle bush, creosote bush, and many varieties of cactus.

Proceed to the Randall Henderson trailhead on the eastern side of the parking lot, in front of the visitor's center. Look for the large kiosk with maps of Palm Desert and descriptions of the area's plants and wildlife. Follow the soft, sandy trail east across the desert wash toward the hills. (You can also pick up the trail along the driveway leading to the visitor center, closer to CA 74). At 0.2 miles, the path curves right (to the left is a NO TRESPASSING sign), and continues along the sandy wash. After another 0.3 miles, the trail narrows and passes between two rock walls, then winds up a short but steep hill before it levels and heads southeast. You can also see CA 74 from here, but it's far enough away not to be intrusive. At 1.1 miles, you will come to a trail junction: stay to the left; the path to the right takes you back to the highway. After another brief climb, the trail levels and follows a saddle ridge for about 0.3 miles, then heads

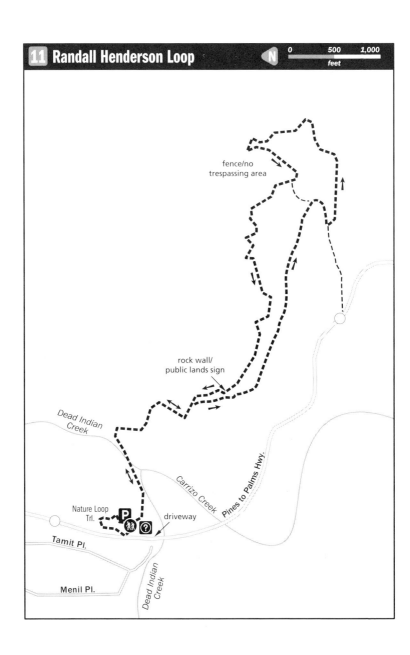

N

0   500   1,000
feet

fence/no
trespassing area

rock wall/
public lands sign

*Dead Indian
Creek*

Carrizo Creek

Pines to Palms Hwy.

Nature Loop
Trl.

driveway

Tamit Pl.

Menil Pl.

*Dead Indian
Creek*

north up wide switchbacks to the trail's high point. Teddy bear cholla cactus are scattered throughout this area. Also known as jumping cholla, they are called teddy bear because their spiny stems appear soft from a distance. You'll also see lots of chuperosa shrubs, creosote bush, and sandpaper plants along this part of the trail.

The trip back down the mountain begins when you reach a sign and a fence blocking public access. Continue on the trail as it loops back down the mountain. Look for the green spiny branches of ocotillo trees, which spike with red flowers in the spring, on either side of the path. As you proceed, look for the green spiny branches of ocotillo trees, which are decorated with red flowers in spring, on either side of the path.

At about 1.8 miles from the trailhead, you'll come to a trail junction. Stay right and continue another quarter mile downhill to the desert floor. At this point, the route crosses a few large boulders: it's easiest to scoot down them on your behind, especially if you're not wearing hiking boots. From here, the trail reconnects with the trail you followed on the way in, and it's another 1.2 miles of flat hiking back to the visitors' center.

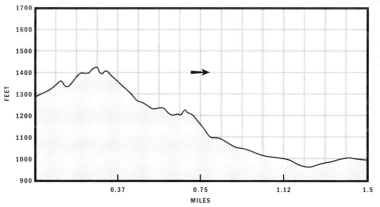

DIRECTIONS: From Interstate 10, exit at Monterey Avenue in Palm Desert and turn right (south). After crossing Palm Canyon Drive (CA 111), continue south as the road becomes CA 74 and drive another 3.5 miles to the visitor center for the Santa Rosa and San Jacinto Mountains National Monument. Turn left and follow the long driveway to the parking lot.

GPS Trailhead Coordinates 11 RANDALL HENDERSON LOOP
UTM zone (WGS 84): 11S
Easting: 0554890.4
Northing: 3725698.4
Latitude: N33.671509°
Longitude: W116.407900°

12 South Lykken Trail

SCENERY: ✿ ✿ ✿ ✿	DISTANCE: *4.5 miles*
TRAIL CONDITION: ✿ ✿ ✿ ✿	HIKING TIME: *2 hours, 15 minutes – 3 hours*
CHILDREN: ✿	OUTSTANDING FEATURES: *desert and valley*
DIFFICULTY: ✿ ✿ ✿	*views, rocky hillsides, Tahquitz Canyon waterfall*
SOLITUDE: ✿ ✿	

The South Lykken Trail is the south half of the 9.5-mile Carl Lykken Trail, which weaves along a series of mountain ridges above downtown Palm Springs. The north and south trails are separated by Tahquitz Canyon, so you can't easily do them as one hike. The South Lykken Trail is a terrific moderate hike featuring wide-open views of the desert valley and a bird's-eye view of Tahquitz Canyon's waterfalls and rock formations. This shuttle hike begins at the south end, follows the trail up a moderately steep hillside, then winds along the mountain ridge past a couple of viewpoints before taking you back down into Tahquitz Canyon at Mesquite Avenue. Expect to see at least a handful of hikers and dogs on this popular trail on any given day of the week.

OPTION: This trail can also be hiked as an out-and-back to the first or second set of picnic tables, or as a 3.2-mile loop by turning right at the first trail split and following the path past Desert Riders Park to Cahuilla Hills Drive, down to Palm Canyon Drive, and then walking south back to the Murray Canyon trailhead.

🚶🚶 Begin by walking west along the dirt road from South Palm Canyon Drive. After about 0.3 miles, the trail narrows and starts to switchback up the hillside to the right. A gradual climb over the next 0.75 miles takes you deeper into the rocky hillsides. You will pass a metal sign for the Carl Lykken Trail on the way up. After about 1 mile, you come to a viewpoint with a few picnic tables and a sign for Simonetta Vista Park. This is a good place to pause for a few minutes and admire the gorgeous views of the Coachella Valley unfurling to the east. It's also a good turnaround point for a moderate 2-mile hike. For the shuttle hike, continue heading north on the trail as it

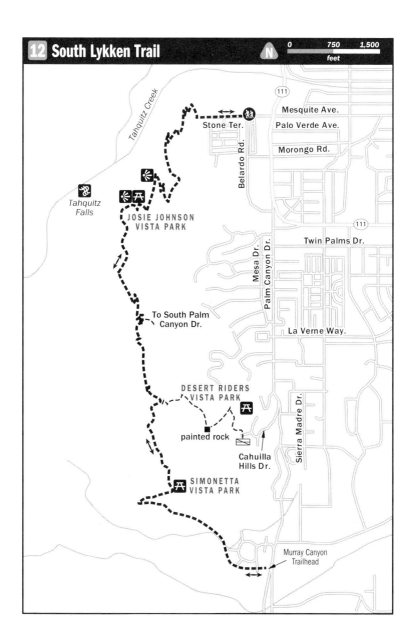

0   750   1,500
feet

Tahquitz Creek

(111)

Mesquite Ave.

Stone Ter.

Palo Verde Ave.

Belardo Rd.

Morongo Rd.

Tahquitz
Falls

JOSIE JOHNSON
VISTA PARK

(111)

Mesa Dr.

Palm Canyon Dr.

Twin Palms Dr.

To South Palm
Canyon Dr.

La Verne Way.

DESERT RIDERS
VISTA PARK

Sierra Madre Dr.

painted rock

Cahuilla
Hills Dr.

SIMONETTA
VISTA PARK

Murray Canyon
Trailhead

snakes along the mountain ridge. After about 1.5 miles, you'll come
to trail split marked by a small pile of rocks, or cairn.

(For a 3.2-mile loop hike, turn right and head downhill to
another viewpoint, known as the Desert Riders Park, with picnic
tables and hitching posts. Then continue past the viewpoint to a rusty
road gate. Pass through the gate into a hillside neighborhood and
follow Cahuilla Hills Drive back to South Palm Canyon Drive.)

To continue on the shuttle hike, take the left (north) trail and
continue heading northwest along the rocky mountain ridge. Views
of Palm Springs and beyond accompany you for the rest of the hike
to the trail's north terminus.After another 0.5 miles of walking,
you'll come to another trail split. Stay left and continue north on the
Carl Lykken Trail. After another 0.5 miles, you will come to another
wide clearing with picnic tables, known as Josie Johnson Vista Park.
This is your last chance to rest and soak up the beautiful views before
heading back down the hillside to Mesquite Avenue. There are usually a few people relaxing here with their dogs or enjoying a picnic

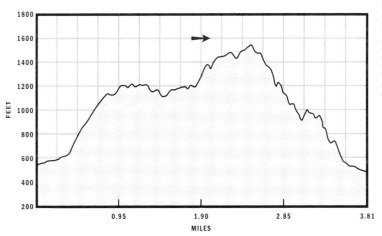

lunch. Hikers who haven't arranged for a shuttle pickup at Mesquite Avenue can turn around here and retrace their route to the Murray Canyon trailhead.

From the picnic tables, the trail winds east briefly before turning north toward Tahquitz Canyon. At about 3.1 miles, be sure to look left for an awesome view of the year-round waterfall in Tahquitz Canyon. From here, the trail heads east, then north again for another 1.2 miles before ending at the driveway for the Tahquitz Canyon Visitor Center. Parking is allowed on Mesquite Avenue, west of South Palm Canyon Drive.

DIRECTIONS: From Interstate 10, take CA 111 south through downtown Palm Springs. Bear right at South Palm Canyon Drive (where CA 111 curves left), and go about 2 miles south, to just beyond Murray Canyon Drive. The trail begins on the right side of the street, just after the housing and condominium complexes give way to wide open fields. Park on Palm Canyon Drive, across from the golf course.

If you're doing the shuttle hike, leave another car near the western end of Mesquite Avenue, just before the entrance to the Tahquitz Canyon Visitor Center off Palm Canyon Drive.

GPS Trailhead Coordinates	12 SOUTH LYKKEN TRAIL
UTM zone (WGS 84):	11S
Easting:	0541095
Northing:	3741820
Latitude:	N33.778719°
Longitude:	W116.545252°

13 Vargas Palms

SCENERY: ✿ ✿ ✿	DISTANCE: *5 miles*
TRAIL CONDITION: ✿ ✿ ✿	HIKING TIME: *2 hours, 30 minutes – 3 hours*
CHILDREN: ✿ ✿	OUTSTANDING FEATURES: *palm oasis, sandy*
DIFFICULTY: ✿ ✿ ✿	*wash, desert vegetation, views of windmill farms.*
SOLITUDE: ✿ ✿ ✿	

This flat out-and-back hike crosses a sandy, tumbleweed-covered canyon wash to reach a palm oasis that was damaged by fire. The trail to the oasis is unremarkable, but once there, you will be rewarded with views of the Coachella Valley and a unique desert oasis of palm trees, caves, and a waterfall. The Bureau of Land Management (BLM) leads occasional hikes to Vargas Palms; call (760) 862-9984 or check the BLM Web site, www.blm.gov/ca/palmsprings, for more information. If you do go without a guide, bring a companion, a compass, and plenty of water and sun protection, and heed the NO TRESPASSING signs.

🏃 Begin hiking southeast toward the San Jacinto Mountains along the sandy, unpaved road on the east side of Snow Creek Canyon Road. Soon you will see a cluster of palm trees in the distance at the base of the mountains. This is Vargas Palms, one of several spring-fed palm oases in the area. At 0.4 miles, you will come to another wide sandy path. Cross it and look for a narrow path that forks east. Stay on this trail for about 0.6 miles as it winds south and then east again, toward Vargas Palms. At 1 mile, the route makes a sharp left; after about 200 yards, it heads south along a combination of narrow sandy trails and fire roads for the next 1.5 miles until reaching a large cluster of boulders. It gets confusing here, as different sandy paths branch left and right. Just continue heading south across the wash, directly toward the palm trees, which are easy to keep in sight. Creosote bush, desert lavender, and several varieties of cactus dot the landscape. It's

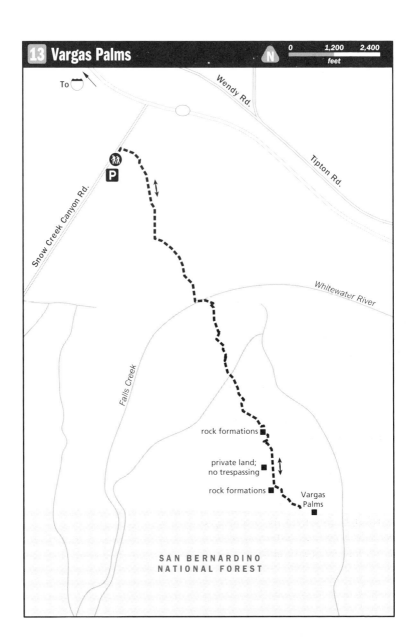

N

0   1,200   2,400
feet

To

Wendy Rd.

Tipton Rd.

Snow Creek Canyon Rd.

P

Whitewater River

Falls Creek

rock formations

private land;
no trespassing

rock formations

Vargas
Palms

SAN BERNARDINO
NATIONAL FOREST

also easy to keep CA III in sight from this trail, as well as the windmill farms that are scattered throughout San Gorgonio Pass.

At 1.75 miles, you'll experience your first real elevation gain as the trail heads uphill and approaches a rocky hillside. The scenery begins to change at this point, leaving behind the wide-open desert landscape for piles of huge gray- and rust-colored boulders.

At 2.2 miles, the main trail ends at a cluster of large rock formations. Take the narrow, sandy trail between the rust-colored rocks (still heading south) and walk uphill toward the palms. The palms loom large and near at this point; if it's windy, the strong whooshing sound of their leaves will dominate the environment. The final 200 yards to the oasis is an easy scramble up more big rocks. From here, pick a boulder to sit on and admire the views of the windmill farms and the San Bernardino Mountains to the north. The oasis is now yours to explore; check out the thick blackened trunks of more than 50 palm trees, peek into the caves, or cool off

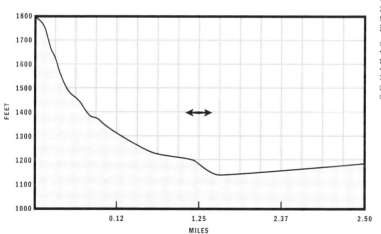

near the small waterfall at the edge of the palm grove. The trees were damaged by wildfires in the late 1990s, but are recovering nicely.

From here, retrace your route to the trailhead. Pay careful attention as you walk and follow the footprints that you left on your way in. Otherwise, you may end up too far south on Snow Creek Canyon Road, a half-mile from where you started. Though CA 111 is in sight for this entire hike, the lack of a defined trail and, in places, high scrub can be disorienting, especially for first-time visitors.

DIRECTIONS: From Interstate 10, exit at CA 111 southbound and go 0.5 miles to Snow Creek Canyon Road. Turn right and go about 0.3 miles toward the San Jacinto Mountains. Park on the side of the road and look for a wide sandy road on the east side of the road.

GPS Trailhead Coordinates	13 VARGAS PALMS
UTM zone (WGS 84):	11S
Easting:	0530469
Northing:	3752386
Latitude:	N33.910966°
Longitude:	W116.669271°

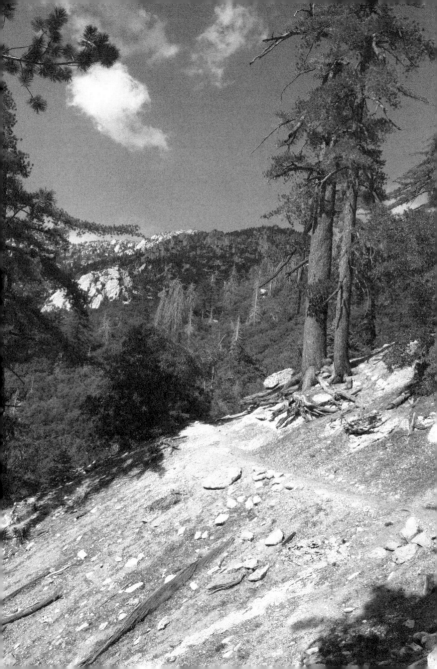

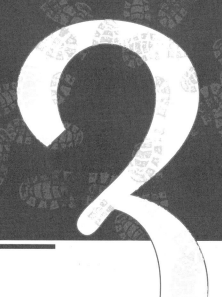

Day Hikes
Other Desert Cities

The striking
mountain
ranges
that
frame
this desert
resort
are
full of
winding
trails
that lead
to natural
palm
groves
year-round
waterfalls
and streams
and
cactus-spiked
desert
terrain

14 Art Smith Trail

SCENERY: 🐾 🐾 🐾 🐾	DISTANCE: 5–8 miles
TRAIL CONDITION: 🐾 🐾 🐾 🐾	HIKING TIME: 3–6 hours
CHILDREN: 🐾 🐾	OUTSTANDING FEATURES: *palm groves, rock*
DIFFICULTY: 🐾 🐾	*formations, panoramic views, bighorn sheep habitat*
SOLITUDE: 🐾 🐾 🐾 🐾	

Named after a local trail builder, this well-maintained trail is a longtime favorite of Palm Springs hikers and equestrians. It begins just off CA 74 in Palm Desert and switchbacks up a hillside before leveling and meandering for several miles past a series of palm oases and views of the Coachella Valley. It totals 16 miles out and back, but many day hikers take it to the second palm oasis or to Magnesia Springs Canyon, and turn back before the trail ends at Dunn Road, a vehicle-restricted road that leads to Cathedral City. Its first 1.5 miles were rerouted in 2006 to steer hikers away from a sensitive bighorn sheep habitat; at this writing, local officials were considering closing the entire trail to hikers during the summer months. Check with the Palm Desert Visitor Center, (760) 568-1441, or the Bureau of Land Management, (760) 862-9984, for updates.

OPTION: This can also be a moderate 4- or 5-mile out-and-back hike to the first series of palm oases.

🚶🚶 Look for the trailhead at the far north corner of the parking lot. You will see a sign for the Art Smith Trail and a map of the Palm Springs area trail system. Begin walking north past the sign along the sandy wash. After 100 yards or so, you will come to a sign indicating that Dead Indian Canyon, a 3-mile out-and-back trail, is closed from January 1–September 30. To pick up the Art Smith Trail, follow the base of the concrete levee, which is right of the sign, north along the wash. After a short walk, look for a water tank that sits beyond a chain-link fence with a gate. Make a sharp left just before the gate and follow the south side of the fence west toward

N

0   1,250   2,500
feet

Pines to Palms Hwy.

Buckhorn Trl.

Kiva Dr.

Bighorn
Country Club

Jaguar Way

Metate Pl.

Menil Pl.

Netas Dr.

Sivat Dr.

Suuwat Way

Tekis Pl.

rock
formations

Grapevine Creek

Tepin Way

small clearing/
rock formations

first palm
oasis

Bridge

Ebbens Creek

the hillside. There is no real trail at this point; you are just walking across a wash of cracked, layered mud that has dried in stages. After 0.4 miles, look for a signpost and a narrow dirt trail winding up the hillside just beyond it. Follow the trail up the hill past desert lavender, sage, creosote bush, and barrel and cholla cactus. You can still see and hear noise from CA 74 as you ascend, but every step gets you farther away from civilization. At 0.7 miles, the path levels and passes a small clearing marked by rock formations; this is a good spot for kids to explore, though they won't have much patience for the remaining shadeless 7 miles of trail. From here, the trail dips north into the canyon and provides views of the strangely green Bighorn Country Club and golf course to the northeast. The trail continues for the next mile in easy switchbacks along the mountain ridge, past a few small boulder-strewn viewpoints overlooking the valley. You will begin to see more cacti, aloe, and other desert plants on either side of the trail.

At 1.5 miles, the Art Smith Trail connects with the 8-mile Hopalong Trail, a recent addition to the desert hiking system that leads to Homme-Adams Park in Palm Desert and the Bump and Grind Trail in Rancho Mirage. Continue straight on the Art Smith

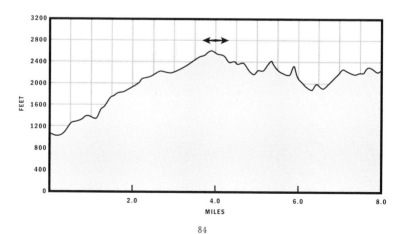

Trail (the Hopalong Trail veers right) as it follows the mountain ridge west. At about 2 miles, the trail crosses a flat clearing dotted with rock formations, then ascends a small hillside to a view of a small California fan-palm oasis. Follow the trail to the right of the palms, then look for an unsigned post and go left up a short, steep hill. Continue another 0.5 miles along a wide, sandy trail to a series of three more palm groves and fine views of the valley framed by rocky hillsides. At about 3 miles, you will reach a small clearing with boulders for sitting and more great views of the valley. This is a good turnaround point for those looking for a short day hike. Or you may continue another 2.2 miles to Magnesia Springs Canyon, home to another shady palm oasis that makes a good spot to stop for lunch. From Magnesia Springs Canyon, the Art Smith Trail winds north-west until it ends at Dunn Road, a no-vehicles road that links with the Hahn Buena Vista and Vandeventer trails, two strenuous trails popular with mountain bikers, which lead into the Indian Canyons. Dunn Road heads north and eventually ends at a wash near Cathedral City Cove, but it's not recommended that hikers follow this path because of private-land issues.

DIRECTIONS: From Interstate 10, exit at Monterey Avenue in Palm Desert and drive south several miles. After crossing Palm Canyon Drive (CA 111), continue south, now on SR 74, past Thrush Road, for about 4 miles. Look for the small Art Smith Trail parking lot on the right, just past the visitor center for the Santa Rosa and San Jacinto Mountains National Monument. The Palm Desert Visitor Center, 72-567 Highway 111, has a good hiking map of the area and is a source for updates on trail conditions and reroutes.

GPS Trailhead Coordinates	14 ART SMITH TRAIL
UTM zone (WGS 84):	11S
Easting:	3725563
Northing:	0554846
Latitude:	N33.668960°
Longitude:	W116.41025

15 Big Morongo Canyon Trail

SCENERY: 🐾 🐾 🐾 🐾	DISTANCE: 2–9 miles
TRAIL CONDITION: 🐾 🐾 🐾 🐾	HIKING TIME: 2–4 hours
CHILDREN: 🐾 🐾 🐾 🐾	OUTSTANDING FEATURES: ancient rocks,
DIFFICULTY: 🐾 🐾	unique desert wetland, bighorn sheep, 240 species
SOLITUDE: 🐾 🐾 🐾	of birds

This moderate balloon hike is a good introduction to Big Morongo Preserve, a 29,000-acre desert oasis of marshes, ridges, canyons, and one of the largest cottonwood and willow riparian habitats in California. The hike begins in a quiet marsh, then heads uphill briefly to a saddle ridge before dipping into Big Morongo Canyon and following a stream, fed by snow melt from the surrounding mountains, 4 miles to Indian Avenue in Desert Hot Springs. This used to be a popular shuttle hike, but a fence on private property now blocks access to Indian Avenue, and you must turn around at the fence and retrace your route to the parking lot. Dogs aren't allowed in the preserve. If you do this hike in the winter or following periods of heavy rain, expect to make several stream crossings and do some slippery rock scrambling. At an elevation of 2,500, the area tends to be 10 to 20 degrees cooler than Palm Springs and other desert cities.

OPTION: An easy 2- or 3-mile hike can be pieced together on the network of well-marked trails that begin at the entrance kiosk. These trails are mostly flat, and made of sand or recycled materials.

🚶🚶 Grab a trail guide from the kiosk at the preserve entrance and head south on the easy Marsh Trail (actually a boardwalk made of recycled materials). Continue south on the Mesquite Trail from where the Marsh Trail loops back around to the parking lot, then pick up the West Canyon Trail at about 0.4 miles. Take the sandy trail to the right up the hillside. You'll start to see evidence of the 2005 wildfire that swept across the preserve and damaged thousands of its acres. The trails and signs have been restored, but the charred

15 Big Morongo Canyon Trail

N

0   2,000   4,000
feet

DAY OVERNIGHT HIKES

DAY HIKES

part three
OTHER DESERT CITIES

Morongo Valley

62
Pioneer Dr.
East Dr.

West Dr.

San Jacinto St.

Hess Blvd.

Park Ave.

P

nature center

Mesquite Trl.

29 Palms Hwy.

Matzene Dr.

Canyon Trl.

Big Morongo Creek

BIG MORONGO REGIONAL PARK

62

2-mile signpost

62

Devils Garden

29 Palms Hwy.

Kolbe Rd.

Worsley Rd.

Indian Ave.

Mission Creek

BIG MORONGO CANYON

Colorado River Aqueduct

skeletons of scrub oak trees dot the landscape on either side of the trail. At about 1 mile from the parking lot, the West Canyon Trail ends and meets up with the main Canyon Trail. Follow it to the right (south) as it descends gradually into the canyon, flanked on either side by fields of creosote bush, willow, alder, and mesquite. You may hear the canyon stream gushing to your left, though the water isn't always visible from the trail. After about 1 mile of meandering south across a wide-open field, the trail crosses the stream and heads due east for about 0.4 miles, then heads south again for the remaining 3 miles. The trail occasionally disappears into brush or sand, but well-placed signposts help prevent serious straying. After passing the 2-mile marker (from the beginning of the Canyon Trail), the trail turns west briefly and hugs the hillside before swerving south again and providing excellent views of the San Jacinto Mountains (snow-capped in winter and spring). From here, it's another 2.5 miles of gradual downhill hiking to a fence that blocks access to Indian Avenue. Retrace your route to the main canyon trail, but instead of turning left on the West Canyon Trail, head straight

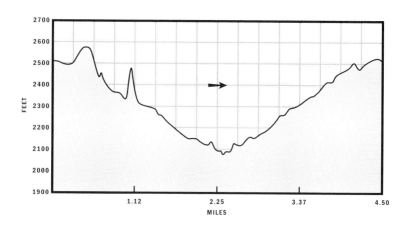

toward the wood fence and follow the Mesquite Trail north. This trail winds past a small nature center and several bird-observation decks with benches. From here, it's another 0.6 miles back to the parking lot. Don't miss the odd arrangement of charred tree branches along the Mesquite Trail near the Robin Kobaly observation deck. It almost looks like they were deliberately placed there as part of a very cool art exhibit. The preserve is managed by the Bureau of Land Management and helped immensely by a strong corps of volunteers known as Friends of Big Morongo.

DIRECTIONS: From north Palm Springs, head west on Interstate 10 and take the CA 62/29 Palms exit. Drive north about 10.5 miles to Morongo Valley and turn right on East Drive. The entrance to the preserve is on the left. Gates are open daily 7:30 a.m. to sunset. For more information, go to www.bigmorongo.com.

GPS Trailhead Coordinates	15 BIG MORONGO CANYON TRAIL
UTM zone (WGS 84):	11S
Easting:	3767847
Northing:	0539665
Latitude:	N34.050568°
Longitude:	W116.569379°

16 Bump and Grind Trail

SCENERY: ✿ ✿ ✿ ✿	DISTANCE: *3.4 miles*
TRAIL CONDITION: ✿ ✿ ✿ ✿	HIKING TIME: *1 hour, 30 minutes – 2 hours*
CHILDREN: ✿ ✿ ✿	OUTSTANDING FEATURES: *expansive views of*
DIFFICULTY: ✿ ✿ ✿	*the desert and mountains; desert vegetation, spring*
SOLITUDE: ✿	*wildflowers*

This popular hike just off CA 111 in Rancho Mirage features a gradual 1,000-foot ascent via switchbacks to a wide-open clearing with spectacular views of the Coachella Valley and San Jacinto Mountains. The trail is well maintained and has several lookout points to stop and soak up the scenery along the way. Don't come here for solitude, especially if it's the weekend. It's very popular with locals as a place to walk dogs and/or get a regular cardio workout.

OPTION: You can also reach this trail via Desert Drive, though you still have to park along CA 111 and walk about half a mile to the trailhead. From Desert Drive, the trail follows a wide dirt-and-gravel path up the mountain and meets up with the Magnesia Falls Trail after about three-quarters of a mile.

🚶🚶 Park (if you can find a space) on Magnesia Falls Drive at Estellita Drive, and find the trailhead near the Rancho Mirage Hiking Rules sign. (Alternate parking is available along Highway 111 at the parking lots for Roy's Restaurant or Provident Bank.) Head north briefly along a flat dirt road, then cross the canyon wash on your right and head straight toward the hillsides. You will be able to see the trail winding up the mountain from here. There are usually quite a few hikers and bicyclists heading up or down the mountain, especially on weekends. This trail is officially called the Mirage Trail, though locals refer to it as Bump and Grind, or the Desert Drive Trail.

After you cross the wash, you'll immediately start climbing up the rocky hillside via easy switchbacks. After about 0.4 miles, the trail

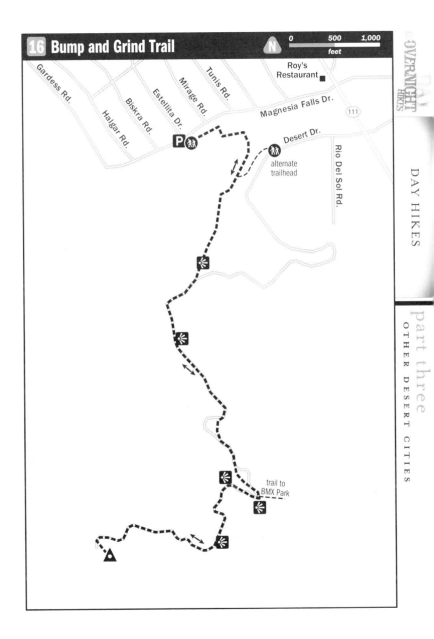

N

0   500   1,000
feet

Gardess Rd.

Halgar Rd.

Biskra Rd.

Estellita Dr.

Mirage Rd.

Tunis Rd.

Roy's Restaurant

Magnesia Falls Dr.

111

Desert Dr.

P

alternate trailhead

Rio Del Sol Rd.

trail to BMX Park

levels and meets up with the wider trail that begins at Desert Drive. Follow the trail right as it winds up the mountain. Soon you'll come to a wide clearing on the left with views of the Coachella Valley. There's no need to stop here, unless you want to, as there are more (and better) viewpoints about every quarter-mile. As you continue up the mountain, you'll notice narrower paths that branch off here and there from the main trail. Most of them eventually just loop back to the main trail. At 0.7 miles, you'll reach another clearing with good views; from here the trail continues to weave uphill along the mountain ridge. For the next half-mile or so, views of the Coachella Valley to the north accompany you as the trail makes a series of long switchbacks. The San Jacinto Mountains (snow-covered and dazzling in winter and spring) weave in and out of sight to the west. Soon you reach another lookout, this one with a view east toward the Salton Sea. Just past this lookout, a trail forks left and heads east over a hillside. This trail connects to other trails within the Palm Desert trail system, including Hopalong Cassidy and Art Smith.

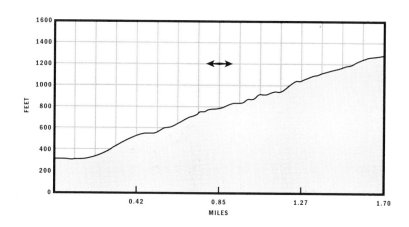

Continue west on the Bump and Grind Trail past another viewpoint that overlooks the lower part of the route. At about 1.2 miles, the trail comes to another viewpoint, this one facing northeast, with big rocks that invite sitting. Look to the east for good views of the golf courses and palm-lined hotel complexes that make up the resort town of La Quinta. The last quarter mile of the trail climbs westward until you reach the trail's clearly designated end—a wide-open clearing with panoramic views of the Coachella Valley and its surrounding mountains. There will likely be a handful of hikers and bicyclists already here enjoying the breathtaking view. The clearing has no rocks or benches for sitting, but there is plenty of room to spread out a blanket or towel and linger for a bit. One Saturday in late December, someone had decorated a lone creosote bush with tinsel and candy canes to celebrate the approaching holidays.

DIRECTIONS: From Interstate 10, take the Monterey Avenue exit and head south toward Rancho Mirage. Make a right on Fred Waring Drive, then a left on Magnesia Falls Drive, just south of Bob Hope Drive. Continue about 0.25 miles to the trailhead on the east side of the road. Limited parking is available on the east side of the road for a few hours a day. Parking is also allowed at Roy's Restaurant at 71959 Highway 111, near Bob Hope Drive, or at Provident Bank, 71991 Highway 111. Parking at the restaurant or the bank will add about a half-mile walk each way to the hike.

GPS Trailhead Coordinates	16 BUMP AND GRIND TRAIL
UTM zone (WGS 84):	11S
Easting:	0554321
Northing:	3732831
Latitude:	N33.734107°
Longitude:	W116.412756°

17 Desert Hot Springs **Loop**

SCENERY: 🌳 🌳 🌳	DISTANCE: *1.2 miles*
TRAIL CONDITION: 🌳 🌳 🌳	HIKING TIME: *45 minutes — 1 hour*
CHILDREN: 🌳 🌳	OUTSTANDING FEATURES: *views of Palm*
DIFFICULTY: 🌳	*Springs and surrounding mountains; desert*
SOLITUDE: 🌳 🌳 🌳 🌳	*vegetation; solitude*

This easy balloon hike begins on the northeast edge of town and follows a flat trail past desert scrub to a small hill that overlooks Palm Springs and the San Jacinto Mountains. A country–club development is planned near the trailhead, but fences clearly delineate the areas under construction. Bring a companion and plenty of water on this shadeless, usually deserted hike.

🚶🚶 Desert Hot Springs doesn't immediately come to mind when one thinks about hiking in the Coachella Valley. But the small, rapidly developing town north of Palm Springs does have a couple of decent hiking trails that afford unique views of Palm Springs and its surrounding mountains and windmill farms. Karl and Ursula Furrer of the Swiss Health Resort have been walking the trails to the north and east of their small hotel for decades with their two dogs and any hotel guest who wants to join them. I joined them one early December morning, when the air was chilly and clear. It had snowed in the surrounding mountains the night before, and we were treated to gorgeous views of white-capped peaks to the south and northwest. While a coat and hat might be necessary in winter, be mindful that Desert Hot Springs hits the triple digits in summer and early fall. Avoid hiking during these months, or go very early in the morning to avoid the crushing heat.

Pick up the flat sand-and-rock trail on the east side of Verbena Drive and follow it east toward a series of scrub-covered hills. The

N

0   450   900
feet

Desert Hot Springs Ln.

Bernardo Way.

Foxdale Dr.

Pomelo Dr.

Pomelo Dr.

Smokewood Cir.

Ambrosio Dr.

Verbena Dr.

San Carlos Rd.

San Felipe Rd.

San Rafael Rd.

San Bruno Rd.

San Ardo Rd.

San Lorenzo Dr.

8th St.

12th St.

Pinto Way

Yucca Dr.

Mesquite Ave.

Swiss Health Resort

6th St.

Sunset Ave.

trail briefly skirts a chain-link fence, then begins a gradual ascent before bearing left and following a wide dirt road away from the country-club development. In late 2006, the area to the south had been cleared for development, but construction had not yet begun.

At 0.4 miles, turn right from the dirt road onto a narrow trail leading due east. Go straight for about 0.3 miles, then veer right up a short hill graced by a small clearing. You won't likely be tired at this point, but take time to stop and admire the expansive views of Palm Springs and the San Jacinto Mountains. The windmill farms visible from here sit in San Gorgonio Pass, one of the most consistently windy spots in the world.

From here, follow the trail west and then south as it descends toward the scrub-covered canyon and loops back to the main dirt road. Turn left at the dirt road and retrace your route past the chain-link fence to the trailhead.

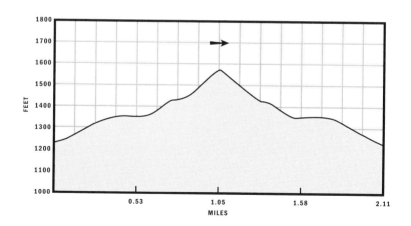

DIRECTIONS: From Interstate 10, take Palm Drive north through Desert Hot Springs. Make a right on 8th Street and continue about 0.5 miles to Verbena Drive. Turn left on Verbena Drive and go about four blocks. Park on the street. The trailhead begins on the east side of Verbena Drive, just north of Yucca Drive.

GPS Trailhead Coordinates	17 DESERT HOT SPRINGS LOOP
UTM zone (WGS 84):	11S
Easting:	0544902
Northing:	3759239
Latitude:	N33.972619°
Longitude:	W116.491924°

SCENERY: 🚶 🚶 🚶 🚶	DISTANCE: *2.2 miles*
TRAIL CONDITION: 🚶 🚶	HIKING TIME: *1 – 2 hours*
CHILDREN: 🚶	OUTSTANDING FEATURES: *views of Palm*
DIFFICULTY: 🚶 🚶	*Springs and surrounding mountains; desert*
SOLITUDE: 🚶 🚶 🚶 🚶 🚶	*vegetation; rock formations, solitude*

This flat out–and–back trail begins on the northeast edge of town and meanders through a quiet canyon studded with boulders and cacti. A country club development is slated to be built near the trailhead, but fences clearly delineate areas of construction. Bring a companion and plenty of water. While a coat and hat might be necessary in winter, be mindful that Desert Hot Springs hits the triple digits in summer and early fall. Avoid hiking during these months, or go very early in the morning to avoid the crushing heat.

🚶🚶 Desert Hot Springs doesn't immediately come to mind when one thinks about hiking in the Coachella Valley. But the small, rapidly developing town north of Palm Springs does have a couple of decent hiking trails that afford unique views of Palm Springs and its surrounding mountains and the windmill farms of the San Gorgonio Pass. Karl and Ursula Furrer of the Swiss Health Resort have been walking the trails to the north and east of their small hotel for decades with their two dogs and any hotel guest who wants to join them. They named one of the trails, enjoyed by many of their guests and friends, the Swiss Canyon Trail, after their home country.

Pick up the flat sand–and–rock trail on the east side of Verbena Drive in Desert Hot Springs and follow it east toward a series of scrub-covered hills. The trail briefly skirts a chain-link fence, then begins a gradual ascent before bearing left and following a wide dirt road away from a country-club development. In late 2006, a wide

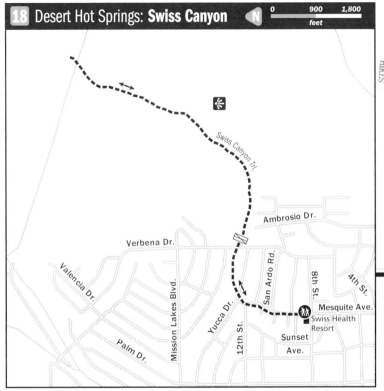

swath of land to the south had been cleared for development, but construction had not yet begun.

At 0.4 miles, you will see a narrower trail leading due east. This is a spur trail, which follows a short loop before rejoining the dirt road. For the Swiss Canyon Trail, continue straight on the wide dirt road as it winds north into the canyon. You are surrounded by desert vegetation and low hillsides. There are also indications that the area may have been used for illegal camping at some point: an abandoned old Buick stripped of its parts, some graffiti here and there. After about a mile, you will reach a cluster of 10-foot-high rock formations, which cast wide shadows across the trail. Follow the sandy trail as it winds between the rock formations to a rock shelf that gives way to open desert landscape. Someone had spray painted "Nirvana" on a nearby rock when I was here last. This can be the turnaround point, or you can climb over the shelf (a moderate scramble that requires decent hiking shoes) and continue another quarter-mile or so into the canyon.

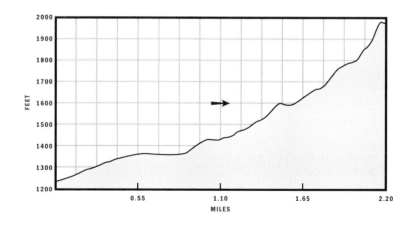

DIRECTIONS: From Interstate 10, take Palm Drive north through Desert Hot Springs. Make a right on 8th Street and continue 0.5 miles to Verbena Drive. Turn left on Verbena Drive and go about four blocks. Park on the street. The trailhead begins on the east side of Verbena Drive, just north of Yucca Street.

GPS Trailhead Coordinates	18 DESERT HOT SPRINGS: SWISS CANYON TRAIL
UTM zone (WGS 84):	11S
Easting:	0544902
Northing:	3759239
Latitude:	N33.972619°
Longitude:	W116.491924°

19 Hopalong Cassidy Trail

SCENERY: ✿ ✿ ✿ ✿	DISTANCE: *2–4 miles*
TRAIL CONDITION: ✿ ✿ ✿	HIKING TIME: *1–3 hours*
CHILDREN: ✿ ✿	OUTSTANDING FEATURES: *sweeping views of*
DIFFICULTY: ✿ ✿ ✿ ✿	*Coachella Valley, desert vegetation, rock formations*
SOLITUDE: ✿ ✿ ✿	

This short but strenuous hike is one of the few on which dogs are allowed (leashed or within 50 feet of owner) in the Palm Springs trail system. It begins at the base of Homme Adams Park in Palm Desert and links with the 8-mile Hopalong Trail, which opened in 2006 as a connector trail to the Art Smith and Bump and Grind trails. Check with the Palm Desert Visitor Center, (760) 568-1441 or the Bureau of Land Management, (760) 862-9984 for updates on trail conditions and closings. You can also pick up a free map of the area's trails at the Palm Desert Visitor Center, just around the corner from Cahuilla Hills Park at 72-567 Highway 111.

🚶🚶 Look for the large TRAIL sign at the northern end of the park and follow the sand trail north as it parallels a wooden fence. When I hiked this trail in early 2007, this was one of the few trail signs I encountered, but a plan was in the works to add more. Soon you'll come to a gap in the fence; go through it, then follow the narrow trail up a steep hill covered in rocks and desert vegetation. At 0.25 miles, the narrow trail ends at a gated fire road. Walk around the gate and continue up the fire road to a scenic overlook with a picnic table, thatched roof overhang, and spectacular views of Palm Desert and the sprawling Coachella Valley. From here, the trail narrows and continues to switchback up the hillside to the west. At 0.4 miles, the path levels briefly, then begins to climb again. You'll see a large water tank below you to the right.

19 **Hopalong Cassidy Trail**

N

0   500   1000
         feet

CAHUILLA HILLS
PARK

P

Desert Cities Baptist
Church parking lot

Vista Pass

Trail to the Cross

fence

fire road gate

Homestead Trl.

fence crossing

Calle De Los Campesinos

Edgehill Dr.

Eagle Rd.

HOMME-ADAMS
PARK

Thrush Dr.

Community
Presbyterian
Church

Cliff Rd.

Pines to Palms Hwy.

Frontage Rd.

At about 0.7 miles, the trail splits, with the left branch continuing uphill to connect with the Trail to the Cross (on which dogs are prohibited). This trail provides stellar views of the valley and San Jacinto Mountains to the west, but it is a steep quarter-mile climb to nowhere—it ends abruptly at a chain-link fence bordering a nearby golf course.

Hikers with dogs will want to turn back at the split or bear right on the Hopalong Cassidy Trail, which travels down the canyon and links with the Gabby Hayes Trail. The Gabby Hayes Trail leads down to Cahuilla Hills Park, at 45-825 Edgehill Avenue in Palm Desert. From here, you can retrace your route to Homme Adams Park (for a total of 4 miles), or arrange to be picked up at Cahuilla Hills Park.

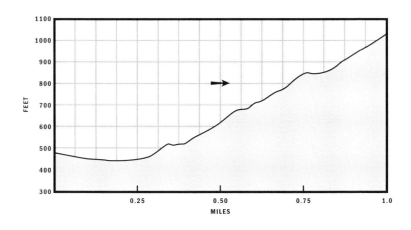

DIRECTIONS: From Interstate 10, exit at Monterey Avenue in Palm Desert and drive south several miles. After crossing Palm Canyon Drive (CA 111), continue south, now on SR 74, to Thrush Road. Turn right, then stay on Thrush as it jogs to the right, then turns left toward the mountains. Follow the road across a small bridge to Homme Adams Park, then turn left and park in the small lot on the right side of the road.

GPS Trailhead Coordinates	19 HOPALONG CASSIDY TRAIL
UTM zone (WGS 84):	11S
Easting:	0555689
Northing:	3729796
Latitude:	N33.706018°
Longitude:	W116.397886°

Day Hikes

Coachella Valley Preserve

4

The strikin

mountai

range

tha

fram

this deser

reso

ar

full o

windin

trai

that lea

to natura

palm

grove

year-roun

waterfal

and streams

and

cactus-spike

deser

SCENERY: ⛄ ⛄ ⛄ ⛄
TRAIL CONDITION: ⛄ ⛄ ⛄
CHILDREN: ⛄ ⛄ ⛄
DIFFICULTY: ⛄ ⛄
SOLITUDE: ⛄ ⛄ ⛄

DISTANCE: *2—4.2 miles*
HIKING TIME: *45 minutes — 2 hours*
OUTSTANDING FEATURES: *desert fan palms, sandy wash, sand dunes, pond*

This mostly flat trail crosses the San Andreas fault and loops around a sandy wash before leading to one of the largest groves of desert fan palms in California and a picture-perfect pond that is home to the endangered desert pupfish. The trail can be shortened to 2 miles round-trip by skipping the Moon Country segment and following the McCallum Trail straight to the palm grove.

OPTION: Many visitors to the Coachella Valley Preserve skip the turnoff for the Moon Country Trail and proceed directly to the McCallum Palms Oasis, then retrace their route to the nature center. This hike, known as the McCallum Trail, is an easy 2 miles round-trip and shouldn't take more than an hour.

The Moon Country Trail is one of several well-maintained trails within the Coachella Valley Preserve, a 20,000-acre property that is home to sand dunes, groves of desert fan palms, and an array of wildlife that includes the rare fringe-toed lizard. Admission is free. Begin your hike under the grove of palm trees off the main parking lot, where you'll find a staffed nature center (open most days), maps, and restrooms. To get to the Moon Country Trail, take the McCallum Trail to the right of the nature center. The sandy trail begins in the shade of palm trees that are believed to be 250 years old. After crossing a couple of wooden bridges, you will come to a fork: follow the McCallum Trail straight (north).

At 0.3 miles, the trail leaves the shade and widens as it climbs a small hill to a junction. The trail to the right leads back to the parking lot. You want to continue straight.

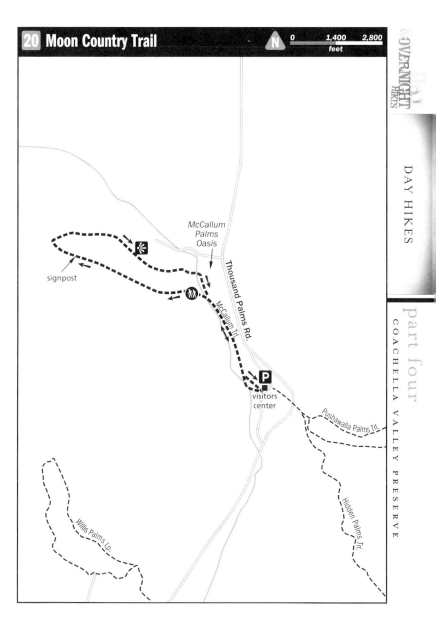

*McCallum
Palms
Oasis*

signpost

Thousand Palms Rd.

McCallum Trl.

P
visitors
center

Pushawalla Palms Trl.

Willis Palms Lp.

Hidden Palms Trl.

Low-lying smoke trees (known for their ash-colored stems) and creosote bushes line the trail. Also here are cattle spinach, a desert weed that sprouts yellow flowers from May to October, and arrow weed. At about 0.5 miles, you'll pass a private home on the right. Continue straight past the driveway, then follow the trail to the left and up a small hill. After another few hundred feet, you will come to another junction. The McCallum Palms Oasis is straight ahead of you. To get to the Moon Country Trail, take the left fork and go up another small hill. You'll see a small sign for the Moon Country Trail; stay left and follow the canyon wash west. The sandy trail becomes a wide canyon wash that here is bordered by brown hillsides and desert scrub. You may think you've wandered off the main trail at times; just keep heading straight (west) and you'll be fine. Look closely at the landscape and you'll see how floods passed through this area at some point: the ground is cracked and many of the bushes lean toward the east. After 2 miles, you'll see a sign post on the right; walk past it and continue north up a narrow, rock-lined trail that

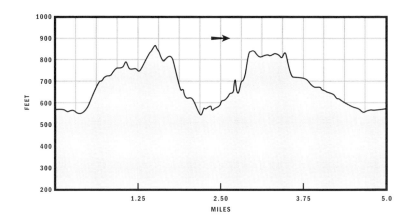

winds up a short hillside. From here, the trail heads back to the east, and you can see the McCallum Palms Oasis in the distance as you head back down the north side of the hill. Now the Little San Bernardino Mountains and Coachella Valley are in full view, as are the flat-top rock formations that dot the landscape north of Thousand Palms Road. At 2.8 miles, you'll reach a lookout point; from here, the trail heads downhill and becomes sandy.

At 3 miles, the trail levels and passes the sand dunes that are a critical habitat for the fringe-toed lizard. Anyone caught trespassing on the dunes will be fined. Follow the trail left as it enters McCallum Palms Oasis. Among the first things you will see as you enter the grove are piles of dry palm fronds; they provide shelter and nesting materials for some of the animals who live in the preserve. Soon the path winds past a pond on the left. This is good place to stop and look for tadpoles and the endangered desert pupfish, a minnowlike fish whose population is dwindling. The trail continues to meander in the shade for another 0.3 miles before reconnecting with the trail that will return you to the nature center parking lot.

Before heading out, take the time to visit the nature center if it's open. Housed in a 1930s log cabin, it has maps, wildlife displays, and a working ice box that is about as old as the cabin.

DIRECTIONS: From Interstate 10, take the Ramon Road exit and head east approximately 8 miles to Thousand Palms Road. Turn left and continue to the preserve's main entrance. The preserve is open daily from sunrise to sunset; it closes during July and August. It's about a 10-minute drive from Palm Springs.

GPS Trailhead Coordinates	20 MOON COUNTRY TRAIL
UTM zone (WGS 84):	11S
Easting:	0563975.6
Northing:	3744163.4
Latitude:	N33.837534°
Longitude:	W116.308567°

SCENERY: 🐾 🐾 🐾 🐾	DISTANCE: *5 miles*
TRAIL CONDITION: 🐾 🐾 🐾	HIKING TIME: *2 hours*
CHILDREN: 🐾 🐾	OUTSTANDING FEATURES: *palm groves,*
DIFFICULTY: 🐾 🐾	*desert and mountain views, Mission Creek*
SOLITUDE: 🐾 🐾 🐾	*earthquake fault*

The Pushawalla Palms Trail is one of several well-maintained trails within the Coachella Valley Preserve, a 20,000-acre property that is home to sand dunes, groves of desert fan palms, and an array of wildlife that includes the rare fringe-toed lizard. It begins near the visitor center and follows the ridge of an uplifted earthquake fault past stunning views of the Coachella Valley down to a large palm grove, then returns via a scrub-covered wash. I like to do this hike in late afternoon, when the sinking sun casts dramatic shadows over the desert and the San Bernardino Mountains. This is an easy-to-moderate hike with an elevation gain of about 300 feet.

OPTION: Instead of looping north at Pushawalla Palms, follow the signs for Horseshoe Palms to the west, just before the entrance to the Pushawalla Palms grove. This heads southwest past Horseshoe and Hidden Palms, then loops north to rejoin the Pushawalla Trail just before the parking pullout. The round-trip total of this loop hike is 4.3 miles.

🏃 Pick up a map of the preserve's trail system at the nature center on Thousand Palms Canyon Road and look for signs marking the start of the Pushawalla Palms Trail on the southeast side of the parking lot. Cross Thousand Palms Road to the official start of the trial. There is a parking pullout at the trailhead, but there was a problem with recurring break-ins here at the time of this writing. Start walking southeast across a wash filled with cacti and brush toward what looks like a low mountain ridge. Follow the signs for the Pushawalla and Horseshoe Palms trails (a signed trail leading to Hidden Palms branches right soon after you begin). After about

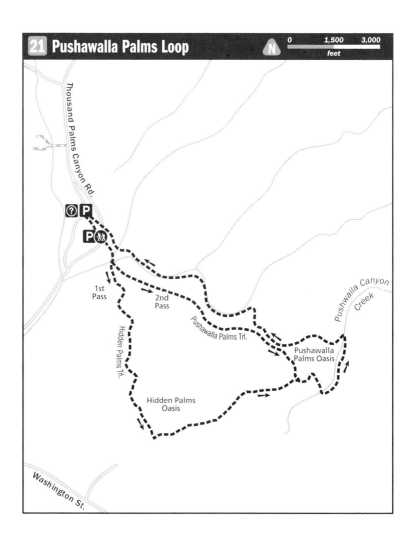

21 Pushawalla Palms Loop

N

0   1,500   3,000
feet

Thousand Palms Canyon Rd.

1st Pass

2nd Pass

Hidden Palms Trl.

Pushawalla Palms Trl.

Pushawalla Palms Oasis

Pushawalla Canyon Creek

Hidden Palms Oasis

Washington St.

0.5 miles, you will reach a flight of wooden steps that lead straight up the fault ridge. At the top, the trail follows the ridge for about 1 mile, past terrific views of the Coachella Valley to the south and the Little San Bernardino Mountains to the north. You are walking along an uplifted edge of the Mission Creek earthquake fault, a branch of the San Andreas fault system. After about 0.5 miles, the Hidden Palms oasis is below you on the right. There are no clearings or resting areas along the ridge, but the entire walk is one big photo opportunity—there is no bad angle. Continue walking east another 0.5 miles or so, until the trail dips back down to the canyon floor. At the bottom, the trail splits. Head right (southeast) to continue down to Pushawalla Palms Trail, following a dry, rock-filled streambed for about 0.3 miles until it becomes a sandy trail that leads to the palm grove. From here, follow the trail north as it skirts the entire palm grove and loops back to the canyon wash. At the trail split near the fault ridge, take the sandy, right-hand path back toward the visitor center. The earthquake fault ridge that you followed on the way in will be on your left. The views are somewhat less interesting on the

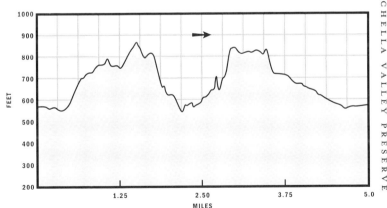

walk back to the nature center, but you will see a variety of desert vegetation, from cacti to desert lavender to creosote bush. A prominent landmark is a tall scorched palm trunk that stands by itself between the wash trail and the fault ridge. From here, it's another mile back to the visitor center.

Before heading out, take the time to visit the nature center if it's open. Housed in a 1930s log cabin, it has maps, wildlife displays, and a working ice box that is about as old as the cabin. If you leave your car in the nature center's parking lot, be sure to pick it up by sunset.

DIRECTIONS: From Interstate 10, take the Ramon Road exit east of Palm Springs and head east approximately 8 miles to Thousand Palms Canyon Road. Turn left and continue to the main entrance. The preserve is free and open from sunrise to sunset daily; it closes during July and August. It's about a 10-minute drive from Palm Springs.

GPS Trailhead Coordinates	21 PUSHAWALLA PALMS LOOP
UTM zone (WGS 84):	11S
Easting:	N33° 50.2773'
Northing:	W116° 18.5062'
Latitude:	N33.835389°
Longitude:	W116.306161°

22 Willis Palms Loop

SCENERY: ✦ ✦ ✦
TRAIL CONDITION: ✦ ✦ ✦ ✦
CHILDREN: ✦ ✦ ✦ ✦
DIFFICULTY: ✦ ✦
SOLITUDE: ✦ ✦ ✦

DISTANCE: *2-4 miles*
HIKING TIME: *1 to 1.5 hours*
OUTSTANDING FEATURES: *palm grove, desert vegetation, mountain views*

The Willis Palms Loop is an easy hike to a beautiful palm oasis within the Coachella Valley Preserve trail system. The loop requires a moderate scramble up a rocky hillside, but the rest of the route is mostly flat and easy to follow. No dogs are allowed. Traffic noise from Ramon Road and views of electric towers mar the first leg of the hike, but the hike gets more secluded and scenic once it reaches the palm grove.

OPTION: This can also be an easy, flat 2-mile hike by turning around at the western edge of the palm grove and retracing your route to the trailhead.

The Coachella Valley Preserve is a 20,000-acre property that is home to sand dunes, groves of desert fan palms, and an array of wildlife that includes the rare fringe-toed lizard. Admission is free. There are several trails within the preserve; Willis Palms is one of the few that doesn't begin in the main parking lot on Thousand Palms Road.

Look for the trailhead just beyond the gate bordering the parking pullout on Thousand Palms Road. Begin walking northwest along a sandy wash toward the palm grove. At 0.25 miles, you'll come to a fork; bear right and up a small hill. At this point, you're heading north, away from the palm grove, but the trail soon curves back to the south. At 0.4 miles, the trail splits again; head left (south) toward Ramon Road and continue 0.2 miles toward the palm oasis. Look for a small signpost to the southwest and follow the trail as it winds along the south side of the palm grove. At 0.9 miles, you'll reach the

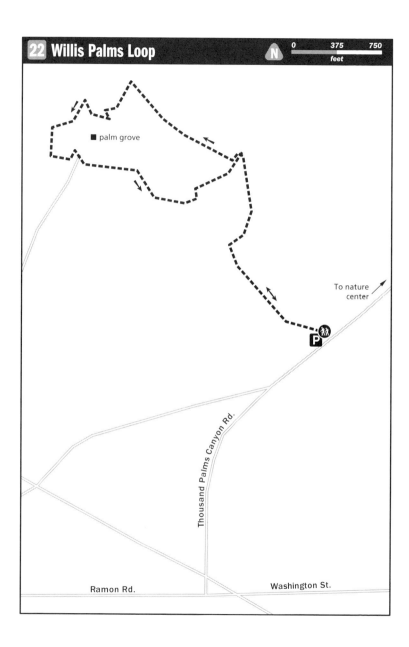

N

0   375   750
                    feet

palm grove

To nature
center

P

Thousand Palms Canyon Rd.

Ramon Rd.

Washington St.

far western end of the grove, marked by a rusty post and a separate sign saying HABITAT RESTORATION IN PROGRESS. From here, you can retrace your route to the parking lot for an easy 2-mile hike, or follow the trail uphill to the cool, protected shade of the palm grove. After exploring the grove, continue on the trail as it heads northwest out of the palm grove, then veers to the right (north), gently climbing a rocky hillside. This part of the trail takes you deeper into the preserve and is the most secluded part of the hike. At about 1.8 miles, the trail loops back and heads south toward the palm grove, following the base of a rocky hill. It reconnects with the main trail at 2.7 miles and heads southeast to the parking pullout.

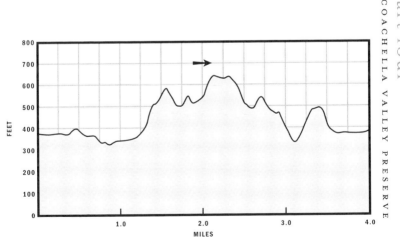

DIRECTIONS: From Interstate 10, take the Ramon Road exit and head east approximately 8 miles to Thousand Palms Road. Turn left and continue about 0.4 miles until you see a small sign for the Coachella Valley Preserve. Park in the small pullout on the left (west) side of the road. Maps and restrooms are available at the nature center, which you'll find on Thousand Palms Road about 1 mile ahead.

GPS Trailhead Coordinates	22 WILLIS PALMS LOOP
UTM zone (WGS 84):	11S
Easting:	0562580
Northing:	3742645
Latitude:	N33.822159°
Longitude:	W116.322914°

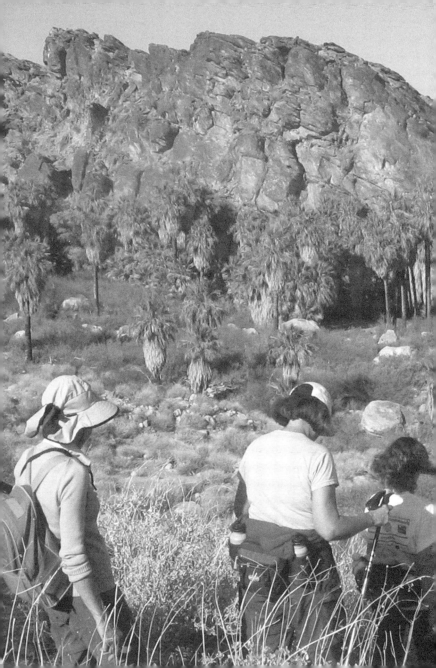

Overnight Hikes

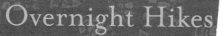

Santa Rosa and
San Jacinto Mountains

5

The striking
mountain
range
that
frame
this desert
resort
are
full of
winding
trail
that lead
to natural
palm
grove
year-round
waterfall
and streams
and
cactus-spiked
desert
terrain

23 Black Mountain Road Trail

SCENERY: 🐾 🐾 🐾 🐾
TRAIL CONDITION: 🐾 🐾 🐾 🐾
CHILDREN: 🐾 🐾
DIFFICULTY: 🐾 🐾 🐾
SOLITUDE: 🐾 🐾 🐾

DISTANCE: *12 miles*
HIKING TIME: *5–6 hours*
OUTSTANDING FEATURES: *gorgeous mountain views, manzanita, desert vegetation, fire lookout*

This hike begins about 5 miles outside of Idyllwild Village and follows a wide fire road up a relentless 2,400 feet to a campground and lookout tower with panoramic views of the San Jacinto and San Bernardino mountains and San Gorgonio Pass. Some hikers prefer to do this hike in early spring, when the road is still closed to vehicular traffic and they have the views all to themselves. Pick up a wilderness permit at the Idyllwild Ranger Office, even for a day hike. The Forest Service staff can also give you updated information on road and campground closures and conditions.

OPTION: The road is open to four-wheel-drive vehicles in the late spring and summer, though you will need an Adventure Pass to leave your car anywhere within the forest boundaries. You may drive to Boulder Basin Campground, and use that for a base to explore other nearby trails, including Fuller Ridge and the Pacific Crest Trail. Keep in mind that Boulder Basin closes for the winter season and often doesn't reopen until mid-May.

🥾 Pick up the dirt fire road just beyond the U.S. Forest Service sign for Black Mountain Road/Fuller Ridge Trail on the north side of Hwy. 243. The elevation gain kicks in immediately on this hike, which quickly envelopes you in a peaceful wilderness setting. It is almost entirely uphill until you reach Boulder Basin Campground. You will pass several unsigned trail splits; stay on the wide, winding fire road to reach Black Mountain Trail; the road is paved in some spots, but mostly packed dirt. Expect to see groves of oaks, pines, and scrub on the lower part of the trail. The pine forest gets denser and more beautiful the farther in you get. At about 4.1 miles, you

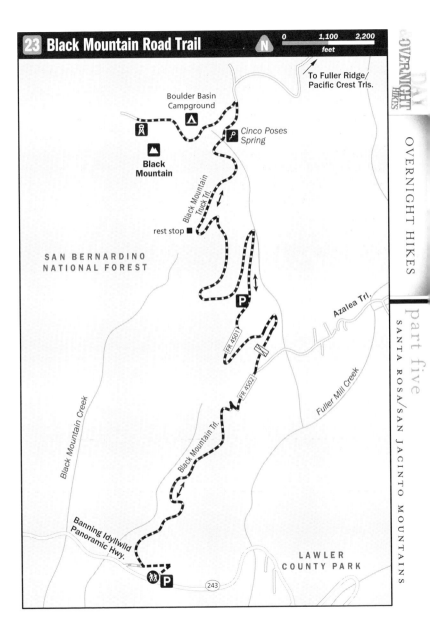

N

0   1,100   2,200
feet

To Fuller Ridge/
Pacific Crest Trls.

Boulder Basin
Campground

Cinco Poses
Spring

Black
Mountain

Black Mountain
Truck Trl.

rest stop

SAN BERNARDINO
NATIONAL FOREST

FR 4S01

Azalea Trl.

FR 4S02

Black Mountain Creek

Black Mountain Trl.

Fuller Mill Creek

Banning Idyllwild
Panoramic Hwy.

LAWLER
COUNTY PARK

(243)

will reach an unmarked clearing on the left. This is a staging area for the U.S. Forest Service; no camping is allowed. Fringed by towering pines and large logs, it is a scenic place to stop and rest before continuing the remaining 2 miles to Black Mountain.

At about 5.3 miles, make a sharp left and follow the road about 0.25 miles past Boulder Basin Campground to its end. Take the paved path to the lookout tower, which is staffed by volunteers from May to September. If it's open, you are welcome to climb up the tower and enjoy the panoramic views and learn about fire prevention from the volunteers. On a clear day, you can see the Santa Rosa Mountains, San Jacinto Peak, San Gorgonio Pass, and even the Pacific Ocean. From here, you can retrace your route to the highway, or set up camp at Boulder Basin and explore the other trails within the San Jacinto Mountains the next day.

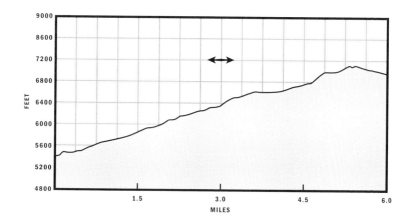

DIRECTIONS: From Interstate 10, take the exit for Idyllwild and CA 243 and follow it CA 243south up the mountain for about 20 miles. About 2 miles past the Vista Grande Ranger Station, look for a sign for Black Mountain Road and turn left into the parking pullout. The road is usually closed to cars from November through April but is open for hiking year-round.

GPS Trailhead Coordinates	23 BLACK MOUNTAIN ROAD TRAIL
UTM zone (WGS 84):	11S
Easting:	0525754.0
Northing:	3734623.2
Latitude:	N33.753112°
Longitude:	W116.721928°

24 Cactus Springs Trail

SCENERY: ✿ ✿ ✿	DISTANCE: *9 miles*
TRAIL CONDITION: ✿ ✿ ✿	HIKING TIME: *5–6 hours*
CHILDREN: *Not recommended*	OUTSTANDING FEATURES: *mountain views,*
DIFFICULTY: ✿ ✿ ✿	*manzanita, desert vegetation, seasonal stream*
SOLITUDE: ✿ ✿ ✿	

This moderately challenging hike is the primary access route into the starkly beautiful Santa Rosa Wilderness. It zigzags through fields of sentinel yuccas and cacti, past an abandoned limestone quarry, and across a shaded creek—deep into the arid desert wilderness. The first 2.3 miles to Horsethief Creek are mostly downhill, but then the trail heads out of the canyon for a rough and steep 4.5 miles to Cactus Springs (which is always dry) with views of the 6,500-foot pine-covered Martinez Mountain. Camp overnight at the year-round Pinyon Flats Campground ($8 a site; first come, first served) across the street from the trailhead, or set up camp near Horsethief Creek and finish the hike the next day; the last 4.5 miles have little shade and can be very hot from April to October. For updates on camping conditions in the area, contact the Santa Rosa and San Jacinto National Monument Visitor Center at (760) 862-9984.

OPTION: Dog owners and day hikers can take this trail to Horsethief Creek, rest a bit in the shade, and then head back, which makes for a moderate 5-mile out-and-back hike.

🚶 Look for the trailhead sign at the east end of the parking lot and follow a wide dirt road east beyond the sign for Cactus Springs. An unsigned trail to the left leads to an Elks Lodge. Bikes aren't allowed here, but dogs and horses are. The first 2.5 miles are good for dogs, but after that the path gets rough and steep with many loose rocks. Continue on the dirt road about 0.2 miles to another sign for Cactus Springs. This marks the official start of the trail. If you

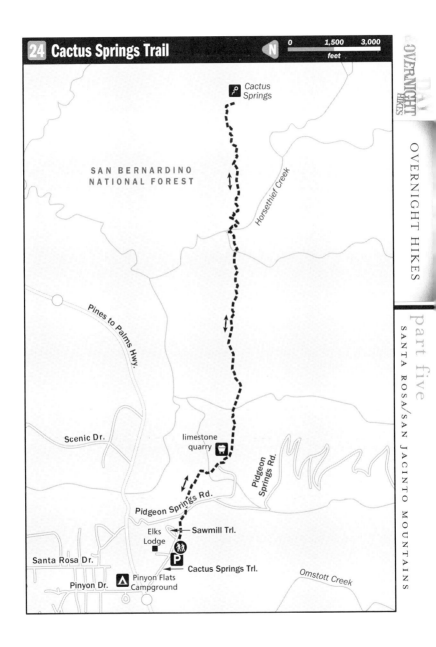

24 **Cactus Springs Trail**

OVERNIGHT HIKES

DAY OVERNIGHT HIKES

OVERNIGHT HIKES

part five
SANTA ROSA/SAN JACINTO MOUNTAINS

0   1,500   3,000
        feet

N

Cactus Springs

SAN BERNARDINO
NATIONAL FOREST

Horsethief Creek

Pines to Palms Hwy.

Scenic Dr.

limestone
quarry

Pidgeon Springs Rd.

Pidgeon Springs Rd.

Elks
Lodge

Sawmill Trl.

P

Cactus Springs Trl.

Santa Rosa Dr.

Pinyon Flats
Campground

Pinyon Dr.

Omstott Creek

continue straight on the dirt road, it will lead you a strenuous
9 miles up Sawmill Road to the base of Toro Peak.

For this hike, take the loose dirt trail to the left as it heads down
into the canyon and past another trail sign and sign-in register. This
is also where you should fill out a self-issued wilderness permit if you
plan on camping overnight. The next 2 miles are an up-and-down
trek (mostly down) past manzanita, desert sage, cacti, and other vegetation. There is little shade and few places to stop along this part of
the trail. After about 0.5 miles, an old limestone quarry and its rusty
machinery will come into view. The trail takes you farther down into
the canyon, then up and around to the quarry, where you can examine the white and pink crystallized dolomite rocks that were mined
here.

Continue east on the trail as it heads past the quarry and a
small clearing to a sign that warns hikers to beware of "hazardous
conditions beyond this point." Most likely, the sign is referring to
the loose gravel trail that can be quite slippery after a rainfall. Hikers
should also beware that this is rattlesnake country; keep an eye out
for them as you walk, especially during the hot weather months.

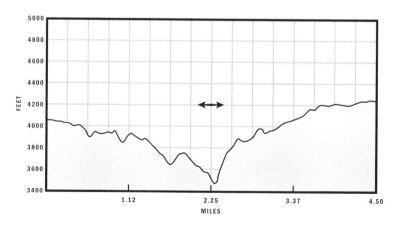

At 1.8 miles, Horsethief Creek comes into view below you to the left, and it's another 0.5 miles, downhill, to the creek. There are a few large rocks, fallen logs, and cottonwood trees at the crossing, marking the best place along the trail to rest and rehydrate or pitch a tent and spend the night. As the story goes, the creek got its name because nineteenth-century horse thieves used to hide the animals in this densely wooded area before driving them to the cities to sell.

From here, the trail heads uphill for a steep quarter-mile to a mountain ridge, then follows a dry canyon wash for about 2 miles. Cactus Springs is supposedly located 100 yards or so to the north of the trail, though there were no signs of a spring when I did this hike in early April. The area really doesn't invite lingering, but stop for a moment to take in the solitude and desolate desert wilderness and you'll begin to appreciate why the horse thieves liked to hide out here.

Keep in mind that the trip back will be tougher than the hike in—the elevation gain between Horsethief Creek and the trailhead is about 900 feet. Bring plenty of water and sunscreen. Though this is a popular and well-known trail, it doesn't tend to get much traffic; I only saw two horseback riders when I hiked it on a Saturday morning.

DIRECTIONS: From CA 111 in Palm Desert, head south on CA 74 for about 14 miles to Pinyon Flat Campground (from Idyllwild, it's about a 26-mile drive). Turn left (south) at the sign for Sawmill Road, directly across from the Pinyon Flats Campground, follow it about 0.5 miles, and then make a left into the parking lot just before the Waste Transfer Station. Park in the large lot and look for the sign for the Cactus Springs Trail at the lot's eastern edge.

GPS Trailhead Coordinates	24 CACTUS SPRINGS TRAIL
UTM zone (WGS 84):	11S
Easting:	0551076.6
Northing:	3715518.9
Latitude:	N33° 34.7939'
Longitude:	W116° 27.0281'

SCENERY: 🌵 🌵 🌵 🌵	DISTANCE: *6.4 miles*
TRAIL CONDITION: 🌵 🌵 🌵	HIKING TIME: *3–4 hours*
CHILDREN: 🌵	OUTSTANDING FEATURES: *mountain views,*
DIFFICULTY: 🌵 🌵 🌵	*manzanita, views of Palm Springs and the Coachella*
SOLITUDE: 🌵 🌵 🌵 🌵	*Valley*

This quiet out–and–back hike is one of my favorites in the Palm Springs area. It's easy to follow, provides a moderate cardio workout, and is marked by thick groves of manzanita and gorgeous views of both mountain and desert. It starts out traversing privately owned pastures, switchbacks up a mountain for 1.5 miles, crosses the Pacific Crest Trail, and then heads downhill for a mile to Cedar Springs, a beautiful and shaded campsite that invites lingering. The hike can be done year–round, though the best times are spring and early fall.

🚶 Walk through the unlocked gate on the right side of Morris Ranch Road and follow a dirt road northeast toward the mountains. Be mindful that this road passes through parcels of private property for the first mile, so be respectful of the NO TRESPASSING signs and the fences on either side of the trail. Dogs are allowed but should be kept on a leash for the first mile. At 0.25 miles, you will come to another unlocked gate; walk through it and continue following the dirt road up a gradual incline. The road starts to get narrower and filled with loose rocks at this point, and it's well shaded by dense oaks and pines. Soon you'll come to a large sign indicating that Cedar Springs is 3 miles ahead. The road continues gently uphill past desert lavender, sage, manzanita, yucca, and paddle cactus.

At 0.8 miles, you'll pass two old picnic tables nestled in an attractive clearing. Continue walking as the road turns into a trail and veers east and heads through dense forest before ascending the mountainside in long switchbacks. Just before you reach the 1-mile

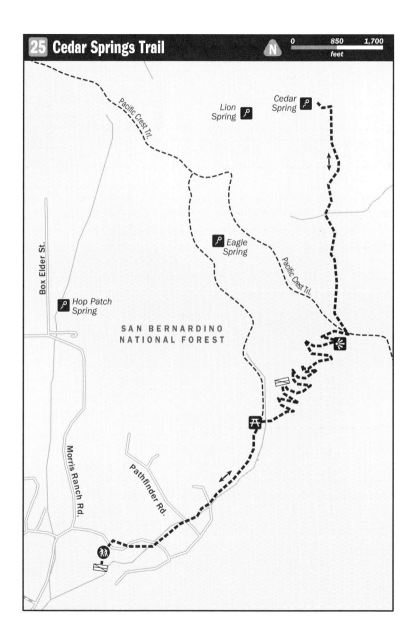

N

0   850   1,700
feet

Pacific Crest Trl.

Lion
Spring

Cedar
Spring

Eagle
Spring

Box Elder St.

Hop Patch
Spring

Pacific Crest Trl.

SAN BERNARDINO
NATIONAL FOREST

Morris Ranch Rd.

Pathfinder Rd.

point, you'll come to a sign for the Pacific Crest Trail (1.5 miles from here) and Cedar Springs (2.5 miles). The next 1.5 miles are a steady uphill climb accompanied by terrific views of Garner Valley and the San Jacinto Mountains. The trail skirts a seasonal stream before the switchbacks begin, though it was only a trickle when I visited after a drier-than-usual winter.

At 1.2 miles, you'll pass through the last of the unlocked gates; from here, the trail continues switchbacking up the mountainside. At 2 miles, you'll pass a small clearing with a few rocks and wonderful wide-open view of the mountains and the valley. This is one of the few places to stop and rest before reaching the top of the mountain. The trail reaches a saddle at 2.2 miles and meets the Pacific Crest Trail at a four-way junction. There is a natural wood bench shaded by an oak tree tucked into one corner. At this point, elevation 6,800 feet, you've gained 1,400 feet from the trailhead.

To continue to Cedar Springs, take the narrow trail straight as it heads north into the wilderness. The brown and rocky mountainsides of Palm Springs and the Coachella Valley will soon come into view,

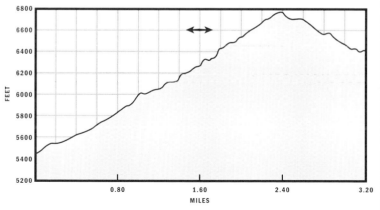

making a nice contrast to the lush green landscape you just left. The next mile is a gradual descent past manzanita, creosote, and other bushes (some of which encroach on the trail) to the inviting back-country campground of Cedar Springs. Set up camp here under the towering pine trees, and spend the rest of the day reading or relaxing by the spring—or use this as a base to explore the Pacific Crest Trail. If you're overnighting, you will need an overnight camping permit (available at the Santa Rosa and San Jacinto Wilderness Visitor Center on Highway 74, or at the Idyllwild Ranger Office). There are no restrooms or trash cans here; you're expected to pack out whatever you packed in.

DIRECTIONS: From the Palm Springs area, take CA III east to CA 74, and then follow CA 74 south about 19 miles to Morris Ranch Road. Make a right and follow the road about 3 miles to a sign for the Cedar Springs Trail on the left. Park on the side of the road, being mindful of the private driveways and NO TRESPASSING signs.

ALTERNATE: The trail is about 10 miles from Idyllwild. Take CA 243 south from town until it meets CA 74 in Mountain Center. Turn left and follow CA 74 about 7 miles to Morris Ranch Road. Make a left and follow the road about 3 miles to a sign for the Cedar Springs Trail on the right. Park on the side of the road, being mindful of the private driveways and NO TRESPASSING signs. Call the San Jacinto Mountains Ranger Station at (909) 659-2607 for more information about overnight camping permits.

GPS Trailhead Coordinates	25 CEDAR SPRINGS TRAIL
UTM zone (WGS 84):	11S
Easting:	0538092.2
Northing:	3723716.5
Latitude:	N33° 39.2463'
Longitude:	W116° 35.3784'

26 Deer Springs Trail

SCENERY: ★★★★
TRAIL CONDITION: ★★★★
CHILDREN: *Not recommended*
DIFFICULTY: ★★★★
SOLITUDE: ★★

DISTANCE: *7.2 miles*
HIKING TIME: *3–4 hours*
OUTSTANDING FEATURES: *mountain views, manzanita, pine forest, rock formations*

This strenuous hike heads up Deer Springs Trail via long switchbacks, then winds 1 mile east up to the top of Suicide Rock, a wide, open clearing with beautiful views of pine-covered mountains and Lily Rock. Easily accessible from downtown Idyllwild and CA 243, this is one of the area's most popular trails, according to the U.S. Forest Service office in Idyllwild. A free wilderness permit is required for this trail; pick one up at the Idyllwild Ranger Station or at San Jacinto State Park Headquarters across the street from the trailhead. Dogs aren't allowed beyond the first 0.25 miles of this trail.

OPTION: Make this an overnight hike by continuing another 2 miles at the junction for Suicide Rock to Strawberry Junction, a flat and shady clearing with 3 primitive campsites and a pit toilet. From here, you can set up camp and the next morning follow the Pacific Crest Trail another strenuous 5 miles up to San Jacinto Peak. From there, it's about an 8-mile hike back down to the Deer Springs trailhead and CA 243. An overnight camping permit is required.

Pick up any of the paths that lead out of the small dirt parking lot; they all funnel into the main Deer Springs Trail. Follow the narrow dirt trail as it heads north up a mountainside via long switchbacks. The first 0.25 miles are a little barren, but you'll start to see canyon live oaks, Coulter pines, and manzanita as you get deeper into the wilderness. At 0.25 miles, the Deer Springs Trail curves right and passes a sign warning that dogs aren't allowed beyond this point. At 0.8 miles, soon after you pass a sign for the San Jacinto

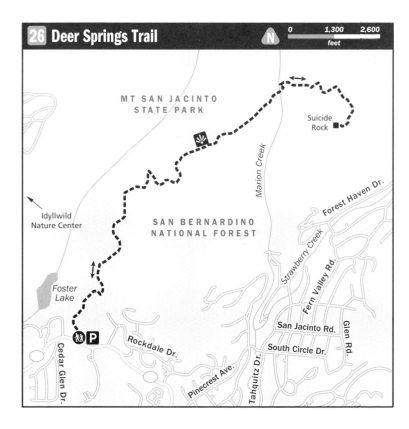

0   1,300   2,600
feet
N

MT SAN JACINTO
STATE PARK

Suicide
Rock

Marion Creek

Forest Haven Dr.

Idyllwild
Nature Center

SAN BERNARDINO
NATIONAL FOREST

Strawberry Creek

Fern Valley Rd.

Foster
Lake

San Jacinto Rd.

Glen Rd.

Rockdale Dr.

South Circle Dr.

Cedar Glen Dr.

Pinecrest Ave.

Tahquitz Dr.

State Park Wilderness, the trail splits. Go left to stay on the Deer Springs Trail; the right path dead-ends at a small viewpoint.

The trail continues to switchback up the mountain for another 1.4 miles before reaching a junction and the turnoff for Suicide Rock. Turn right, then almost immediately left on a narrow shaded trail up the mountain. Pass through the cut in a large fallen tree and continue another mile across Marion Creek to the bleached cliffs of Suicide Rock. The elevation gain between the junction and Suicide

Rock is about 500 feet. Expect to see plenty of purple San Jacinto lupine, manzanita, and buckwheat along this part of the trail. The first half of the day hike ends at the bleached cliffs of Suicide Rock. As the legend goes, the rock got its name after a Native American princess and her unsuitable lover threw themselves off the rock, a la Romeo and Juliet. A more believable piece of data: this is one of the top rock-climbing destinations in Southern California.

After resting and soaking up the panoramic views of Strawberry Valley, you have two options: (1) retrace your route to the parking lot; or (2) retrace your route to the junction, then turn right and climb 2 more strenuous miles on the Deer Springs Trail to Strawberry Junction. Those overnighting should continue another 200 yards to Strawberry Camp, where there are several primitive campsites and pit toilets. The next day, return to Strawberry Junction and continue another 5.5 thigh-burning miles up the mountainside to San Jacinto Peak. An overnight camping permit is required to stay there.

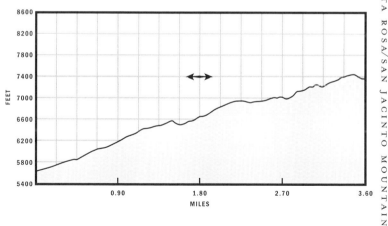

DIRECTIONS: From downtown Idyllwild, drive north 1 mile on CA 243 to the sign for the Deer Springs Trail on the right. Turn right and park in the small dirt lot across the street from the Idyllwild Nature Center.

ALTERNATE: From Interstate 10 in Banning, exit at Idyllwild/ CA 243 and head south up the mountain for about 25 miles. Look for the Deer Springs Trail sign on the left side of the road. Turn left and park in the small dirt lot across the street from the Idyllwild Nature Center.

GPS Trailhead Coordinates	26 DEER SPRINGS TRAIL TO SUICIDE ROCK
UTM zone (WGS 84):	11S
Easting:	0525754.0
Northing:	3734623.2
Latitude:	N33° 45.1751'
Longitude:	W116° 43.3575'

SCENERY: ⛰ ⛰ ⛰ ⛰	DISTANCE: *5–15 miles*
DIFFICULTY: ⛰ ⛰ ⛰	HIKING TIME: *2–6 hours*
TRAIL CONDITION: ⛰ ⛰ ⛰ ⛰	OUTSTANDING FEATURES: *scenic views of San*
CHILDREN: ⛰ ⛰	*Jacinto Mountains and Suicide Rock; pine*
SOLITUDE: ⛰	*forest, sheer rock walls*

This is Idyllwild's most popular hike, according to U.S. Forest Service rangers. A series of moderately challenging switchbacks lead past scenic views of Lily Rock and pine-covered mountains to Saddle Junction, where you can pick up the Pacific Crest Trail or continue all the way to San Jacinto Peak. With a 1,700 foot elevation gain and an easy-to-follow trail, it's a good moderate hike that can be done in a couple of hours.

OPTION: Make this an overnight trip by continuing a mile past Saddle Junction to Skunk Cabbage and Willow Creek. Camp near the stream and continue to the Palm Springs Aerial Tramway the next day (about 4 miles one-way), or explore other trails within the area. You can also reach San Jacinto Peak from here by turning left at Saddle Junction and following the Saddle Junction trail another 5.5 miles to the peak. This should only be attempted by experienced hikers who are prepared with maps and supplies.

🚶🚶 Pick up the trailhead across from the restrooms in Humber Park. Look for the large sign marking the Devil's Slide Trail and follow the trail north into the boulder- and pine-covered wilderness. The trail gets its name from early twentieth-century ranchers who took their cattle to the top to graze before a clear trail was blazed. You'll see why as you begin a steady ascent via long switchbacks on a single-track trail of packed dirt and rocks. The busy parking area quickly fades from sight and is replaced by wide-open views and pine-covered mountains. At 0.7 miles, you'll have to scramble over a large log that blocks the main trail (anyone contemplating bringing

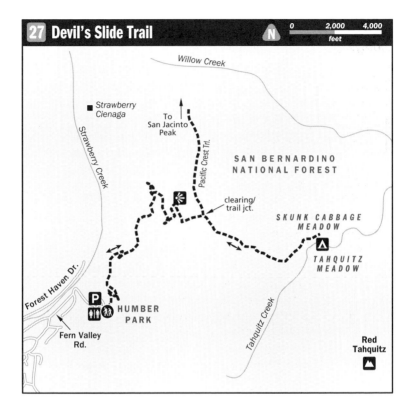

N

0   2,000   4,000
                feet

Willow Creek

Strawberry Cienaga

To San Jacinto Peak

Strawberry Creek

Pacific Crest Trl.

SAN BERNARDINO NATIONAL FOREST

clearing/ trail jct.

SKUNK CABBAGE MEADOW

TAHQUITZ MEADOW

Forest Haven Dr.

HUMBER PARK

Fern Valley Rd.

Tahquitz Creek

Red Tahquitz

children in a back or front carrier should keep this in mind, as it will require removing the child from the carrier). The higher you get, the denser and rockier the surroundings get, with the dirt trail often giving way to natural rock steps as it continues up the mountain.

After about 1.5 miles of uphill hiking, the trail levels briefly and passes a small clearing on the right with a spectacular view of lush green mountains. This is one of the few places for hikers to stop and rest along the trail. Continue another 0.5 miles to a huge boulder and another viewpoint with wide-open mountain vistas. I saw several hikers with dogs on this trail when I hiked it on a late Saturday afternoon. The dogs seemed to be having as much fun scrambling around the rocks and logs as the humans were.

From here, the trail gets narrower and steeper as it switchbacks uphill another 0.25 miles to Saddle Junction. A sheer rock wall hugs one side of the path for awhile just before you reach the saddle. At 2.5 miles, the trail opens to a wide and flat clearing shaded by towering sugar, Jeffrey, and ponderosa pines and strewn with logs and large rocks. This is a great place to stop and rest before heading back or going on to San Jacinto or Tahquitz peaks.

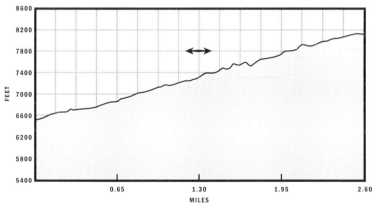

A sign marks the end of Devil's Slide Trail and its junction with several other San Jacinto Mountain trails. Camping is allowed 300 yards from the trail from this point on; most campers prefer to walk another mile to Skunk Cabbage Meadow or Willow Creek, where they can set up camp near a year-round stream. From Skunk Cabbage Meadow, it's about 4 miles to Long Valley and the Palm Springs Aerial Tram. You can also turn left at the junction marking the end of the Devil's Slide Trail and follow the Pacific Crest Trail for about 3 miles, then turn right and continue another mile to campsites in Little Round Valleys. Be sure to pick up an overnight camping permit at the Idyllwild Ranger Station and check with the staff about trail conditions. There is often snow on the ground as late as April or May up here.

DIRECTIONS: **From the center of Idyllwild, follow North Circle Drive to South Circle Drive. At the stop sign, turn right, then make an immediate left onto Fern Valley Road. Stay on Fern Valley Road (being careful not to veer off onto other residential roads) and follow the signs for Humber Park to the parking area. A National Forest Adventure Pass is required to park here (see Backcountry Advice in the front of the book). You also must pick up a wilderness permit for the Devil's Slide Trail at the Idyllwild District Ranger Office, located at 54270 Pinecrest in downtown Idyllwild. Call (909) 382-2921 for more information.**

GPS Trailhead Coordinates	27 DEVIL'S SLIDE TRAIL
UTM zone (WGS 84):	11S
Easting:	0529184.2
Northing:	3735873.4
Latitude:	N33° 45.8587'
Longitude:	W116° 41.1423'

28 Hurkey Creek Trail

SCENERY: 🐾 🐾 🐾	DISTANCE: *2 miles*
TRAIL CONDITION: 🐾 🐾 🐾	HIKING TIME: *45 minutes—1 hour*
CHILDREN: 🐾 🐾 🐾 🐾	OUTSTANDING FEATURES: *year-round*
DIFFICULTY: 🐾	*stream, desert vegetation, mountain views*
SOLITUDE: 🐾 🐾	

This is quite possibly the easiest trail in the Idyllwild area. It's a pleasant walk past desert sage, lavender, manzanita, and a gurgling stream—perfect for children, dogs, and novice hikers. One of the best times to hike the trail is in spring, after a rainy winter, when wildflowers frame the views and the stream is robust with water. Be aware that the trail is also popular with mountain bikers, who pick it up on their way down the mountainside from Keen Ridge.

OPTION: Overnight camping is available at Hurkey Creek and across CA 74 at Lake Hemet. For reservations at Hurkey Creek, call Riverside County Parks at (800) 234-7275. For Lake Hemet, call (951) 659-2680.

Pick up the trailhead on the northern edge of the campground. Walk around the fire road gate and follow the trail north as it parallels Hurkey Creek. From here, it's a flat 1-mile walk past desert vegetation—and with wide-open views of the San Bernardino Mountains—to a small wooden bridge that crosses the creek. Most day hikers turn back here, although you can wander deep into the San Bernardino Forest by continuing on the trail after crossing the bridge, or taking the trail to the left, just before you come to the bridge. Both trails head steeply uphill for several miles, before looping back to CA 74; these trails are more popular with mountain bikers than with hikers.

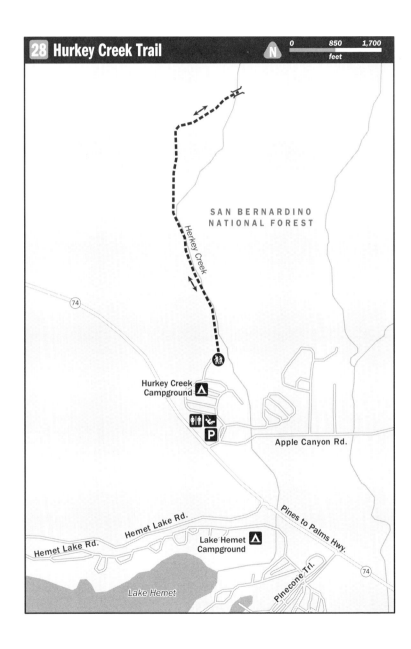

N

0   850   1,700
feet

SAN BERNARDINO
NATIONAL FOREST

Herkey Creek

74

Hurkey Creek
Campground

Apple Canyon Rd.

Pines to Palms Hwy.

Hemet Lake Rd.

Hemet Lake Rd.

Lake Hemet
Campground

74

Pinecone Trl.

Lake Hemet

Hurkey Creek is a stop on the 24 Hours of Adrenaline endur-
ance bike race, which takes place several times a year, in spring and
fall. Hikers will want to avoid this trail during those times. Check the
Web site, **www.twenty4sports.com,** for exact dates.

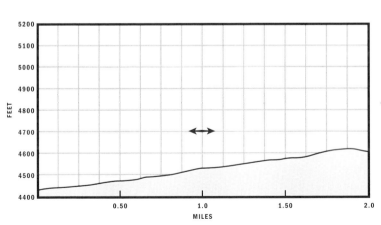

DIRECTIONS: From the Palm Springs area, take CA 111 east to CA 74, then follow CA 74 south about 32 miles to Apple Canyon Road. Make a right, then bear left into Hurkey Creek Campground. Pay a small fee at the kiosk ($2 at this writing), where you can also pick up a map of the Hurkey Creek area, including the campground and trails. and park in the lot beyond the kiosk. The park is open to day hikers from sunrise to sunset.

ALTERNATE: The trailhead is about an 8-mile drive from Idyllwild. Take CA 243 south from town until it meets CA 74 in Mountain Center. Turn left and follow CA 74 about 3 miles to Hurkey Creek Campground. Turn left and head toward the kiosk that marks the entrance to the campground. Pay a small fee at the kiosk ($2 at this writing), where you can also pick up a map of Hurkey Creek, and park in the lot beyond the kiosk. The park is open to day hikers from sunrise to sunset.

GPS Trailhead Coordinates	28 HURKEY CREEK TRAIL
UTM zone (WGS 84):	11S
Easting:	0529584.8
Northing:	3726453.4
Latitude:	N33° 40.7633'
Longitude:	W116° 40.9015'

29 Ramona Trail

SCENERY: ✦ ✦ ✦ ✦
TRAIL CONDITION: ✦ ✦ ✦ ✦
CHILDREN: ✦ ✦
DIFFICULTY: ✦ ✦ ✦
SOLITUDE: ✦ ✦ ✦ ✦

DISTANCE: *8–14 miles*
HIKING TIME: *3–6 hours*
OUTSTANDING FEATURES: *Mountain views, manzanita, ribbonwood, pine forest, desert vegetation*

This well-maintained trail near Lake Hemet is enhanced by beautiful views of the San Jacinto Mountains and a gradual transition from desert landscape to dense pine forest. It begins just off CA 74 and follows several miles of switchbacks up a mountainside covered in pine, manzanita, ribbonwood, and huge rocks to a series of pristine campsites. Day hikers can follow the trail 4 miles to Tool Box Spring Campground, then retrace their route to the trailhead—a moderate out-and-back hike with views that are just as breathtaking on the way back down as when going up. Dogs are allowed on this trail. Start early in the morning if you can, especially in summer, and bring plenty of water and sunscreen any time of the year.

OPTION: You may camp at Tool Box Spring, which has restrooms and fire rings, and use it as a base for exploring the other trails that snake around Thomas Mountain. For a more challenging experience, continue hiking another 2 miles uphill from Tool Box Spring to Thomas Mountain, where there are several primitive campsites (designated by yellow iron posts). The next day, you can take the Ramona Trail back down to your car for a 13.5 mile out-and-back, or continue following a fire road as it winds west, then north, back to Highway 74, for a 14-mile hike. You'll need to have a second car waiting or arrange for a pickup. Thomas Mountain Road is accessible only to four-wheel-drive vehicles, except in icy or snowy conditions.

🏃 Access the Ramona Trail by following the dirt road past a gate on the northwest corner of the parking lot. After 50 yards or so, look for a narrow trail that branches left and follow that another 50 yards to a sign for the Ramona Trail. The single-track trail immediately begins switchbacking uphill past manzanita, ribbonwood, and small

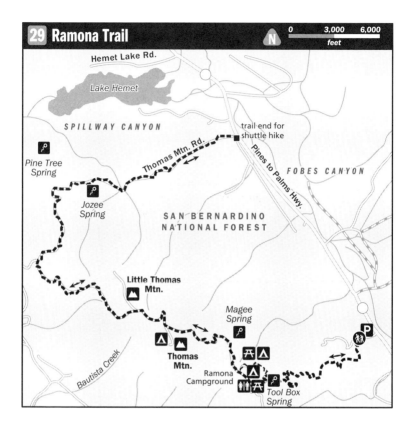

29 Ramona Trail

N

0   3,000   6,000
feet

Hemet Lake Rd.

Lake Hemet

SPILLWAY CANYON

Pine Tree Spring

Jozee Spring

Thomas Mtn. Rd.

trail end for shuttle hike

Pines to Palms Hwy.

FOBES CANYON

SAN BERNARDINO NATIONAL FOREST

Little Thomas Mtn.

Magee Spring

Thomas Mtn.

Bautista Creek

Ramona Campground

Tool Box Spring

clusters of cacti. You'll gain elevation at a steady pace from here on, for a total of 1,700 feet to Tool Box Springs; expect little or no shade on the first mile. The mountain views that make this trail one of my favorites soon appear and stay with you for much of the way to the top. At about 0.6 miles, the trail skirts a small clearing—this is one of the few places to stop and rest along the way. As you approach 1 mile, the sandy trail gives way to larger rocks and gravel and starts to leave the desert landscape behind. After another mile or so of switchbacking, the trail gets shadier, the pine trees that flank it are noticeably bigger and denser, and oak trees dot the landscape. The rocks are also larger and more striking the farther in you go.

At 2.6 miles, the trail is partially blocked by a large fallen tree trunk, but it's fairly easy to climb over. There's another huge log blocking the path at mile 2.8—again it's easy for hikers to manage, but may be a little challenging for cyclists and equestrians who also use the trail. As you near Tool Box Springs, the trail levels for longer stretches and wanders through dense forest before splitting into two separate trails at 3.6 miles. Just before a sign for the Ramona Trail, there is a narrow trail on the right marked by a small post. Take that unnamed trail uphill for about 2 miles to a wide clearing with a few primitive campsites and picnic tables; this trail eventually leads to Thomas Mountain.

For Toolbox Springs Campground, continue straight past several large boulders on the wide trail another 0.3 miles to the camping area, instead of bearing right onto the above-mentioned

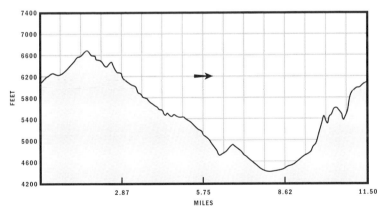

narrow path. You may see some four-wheel drive vehicles at the campground, but I think the hike up the Ramona Trail is a more enjoyable and scenic way to get here. Day hikers can retrace their route to the Ramona Trail parking lot. Overnighters can set up camp and explore Thomas Mountain in the morning. A National Forest Adventure Pass, available at the Idyllwild Ranger Station, is required to park or camp overnight. See Backcountry Advice in the front of the book for more information.

DIRECTIONS: From the Palm Springs area, take CA 111 east to CA 74, then follow CA 74 south about 21 miles, past Pinyon Flats Campground and Morris Ranch Road. Look for a sign for the Ramona Trail to Tool Box Springs, and turn left into a small dirt parking lot. The campsites are run by the San Bernardino National Forest. No reservations or fee are required, but an Adventure Pass is required to park.

ALTERNATE: The trail is about an 11-mile drive from Idyllwild. Take CA 243 south from town until it meets CA 74 in Mountain Center. Turn left and follow CA 74 about 5 miles to the sign for the Ramona Trail. Turn right and park in the small dirt lot. The campsites are run by the San Bernardino National Forest. No reservations or fee are required, but an Adventure Pass is required to park.

GPS Trailhead Coordinates	29 RAMONA TRAIL
UTM zone (WGS 84):	11S
Easting:	0534009.2
Northing:	3720001.7
Latitude:	N33° 37.2727'
Longitude:	W116° 38.0329'

30 San Jacinto Peak

SCENERY: ✿ ✿ ✿ ✿ ✿
TRAIL CONDITION: ✿ ✿ ✿ ✿
CHILDREN: ✿ ✿ ✿
DIFFICULTY: ✿ ✿ ✿
SOLITUDE: ✿ ✿ ✿ ✿ ✿

DISTANCE: *11 miles*
HIKING TIME: *6–7 hours*
OUTSTANDING FEATURES: *panoramic mountain and desert views, pine forest, grassy meadows, ancient rocks*

The first 2.5 miles of this out-and-back hike are a gradual climb through pine forest and grassy meadows to Round Valley Campground. At Wellmans Divide, the trail leads to stunning views of the Santa Rosa Mountains, then soon provides even better vistas of mountains, desert, and ancient rocks—views that stay with you for the remainder of the climb. The total elevation gain of 2,300 feet is gradual but unrelenting. This trail can also done as a day hike, but camping allows you to make the most of Mount San Jacinto State Park and the Palm Springs Aerial Tramway station's offerings.

The San Jacinto Mountains are named after Saint Hyacinth (San Jacinto in Spanish). At 10,834 feet, San Jacinto Peak is the second-highest peak in Southern California.

This hike requires a ride on the Palm Springs Aerial Tramway (at press time, the cost was $21.95 per adult), but the expansive vistas and eventual solitude make it well worth it. The tram whisks you 8,500 feet from the desert floor to Mount San Jacinto State Park, with a corresponding temperature drop of as much as 30 degrees. Camp for a night or two, weather permitting, so you can make the most of trip. If you come to day hike, arrive early and remember that you still must pick up a wilderness permit at the Long Valley Ranger Station. For an advance permit, write to Mount San Jacinto State Park, PO Box 308, 25905 Highway 243, Idyllwild, CA 92549, or phone (951) 659-2607.

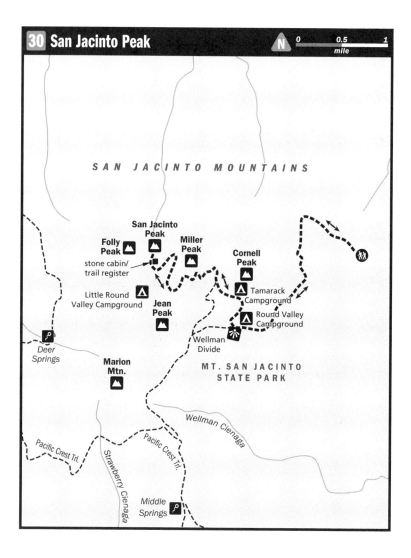

N

0   0.5   1
mile

SAN JACINTO MOUNTAINS

San Jacinto
Peak

Folly
Peak

Miller
Peak

stone cabin/
trail register

Cornell
Peak

Little Round
Valley Campground

Tamarack
Campground

Jean
Peak

Round Valley
Campground

Wellman
Divide

Deer
Springs

Marion
Mtn.

MT. SAN JACINTO
STATE PARK

Wellman Cienaga

Pacific Crest Trl.

Pacific Crest Trl.

Strawberry Cienaga

Middle
Springs

If you hike in the winter or spring, bring waterproof boots and other rain gear. Trail sections that hug rain-swollen creeks are often wet and slippery. Layered clothing is a good idea year-round.

Before heading out, stop at the park office on the ground level of the tramway station for a free map. Head outside and follow the concrete sidewalk as it descends to the valley below. Proceed a quarter mile to the Long Valley Ranger Station and pick up a camping permit (in summer, obtain a permit in advance). At 1.1 mile, you'll come to a sign for Round Valley and San Jacinto Peak. Follow the trail to the left as it skirts a massive fallen tree trunk. From here, it's another mile through dense woodland and between cragged rocks to Round Valley Campground, a flat clearing with 28 sites, pit toilets, and water (though it must be purified before drinking). Set up camp here or continue another half-mile uphill to Tamarack Valley Campground, where there are 12 campsites. Expect to see mule deer, coyotes, black-tailed jackrabbits, and dozens of species of birds in this area. Beyond here expect few hikers.

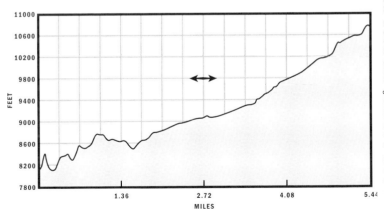

Tired day hikers may be tempted to stop and have lunch at Round Valley, but it's worth it to continue on the main trail another mile to Wellmans Divide, where there are exquisite views and large rocks that invite sitting.

If you're camping, start Day Two by leaving Round Valley and returning to the main trail as it heads southwest toward Wellmans Divide, a small boulder-strewn clearing at an elevation of 9,700 feet. From here, look east for a view of Tahquitz Peak, the Santa Rosa mountain range, and even the Salton Sea. This is also a jumping off point for the Saddle Junction Trail.

Leaving Wellmans Divide, the trail dips north into a rock-strewn pine forest for about a mile, then leaves the forest and follows a manzanita-covered mountain ridge almost the rest of the way to San Jacinto Peak.

After nearly 3 steadily uphill miles, the trail turns sharply to the left and ends just below the peak's summit. Here, you'll find a small stone shelter, built by the California Conservation Corps (CCC) in 1935, which contains bunk beds, a stove, and (usually) the trail register. Anyone can use the cabin.

From the stone cabin, it's a 100-yard climb up a pile of boulders (keep to the left when in doubt) to the peak. A small brown sign atop the highest rock marks the summit. From here, you'll have views of Mount San Gorgonio, the San Bernardino Mountains, the entire Coachella Valley, and even the Pacific Ocean and Inland Empire on a clear day. The naturalist John Muir called it "the most sublime spectacle to be found anywhere on this earth."

The rocky and windy conditions at the summit make camping here difficult, though some hardy souls have attempted it. There are tales of people hiking down the peak at 3 a.m. to take shelter in the stone hut because they couldn't tolerate the cold and strong winds. No matter where you choose to camp, though, the view from the summit is likely one of the best you'll ever experience.

The return trip to Round Valley Campground is an easy downhill trek of 3.5 miles; just make sure you allow for plenty of time to get there before dark. Start Day Three by exploring the woods around Round Valley before retracing your route to the tramway station.

DIRECTIONS: From Interstate 10, take CA 111 south toward Palm Springs and go 8 miles to Tramway Road. Turn right onto Tramway Road and follow it about 4 miles to the Palm Springs Aerial Tramway's Valley Station. Park in the lot. Starting at 10 a.m., Monday through Friday, and at 8 a.m. on weekends and holidays, tramway cars depart at least every half hour. The last tram car departs at 10 p.m. The tramway is typically closed for maintenance in September. For more information call (760) 325-1391.

GPS Trailhead Coordinates	30 SAN JACINTO PEAK
UTM zone (WGS 84):	11S
Easting:	0533393
Northing:	3741713
Latitude:	N33° 48' 54"
Longitude:	W116° 38' 21"

31 South Ridge Trail

SCENERY: ☆ ☆ ☆ ☆ ☆
TRAIL CONDITION: ☆ ☆ ☆ ☆
CHILDREN: ☆
DIFFICULTY: ☆ ☆ ☆ ☆
SOLITUDE: ☆ ☆

DISTANCE: *7–11 miles*
HIKING TIME: *4–5 hours*
OUTSTANDING FEATURES: *Tahquitz Peak,
historic fire lookout, views of Palm Springs and the
Coachella Valley, dramatic rock formations*

*This strenuous hike near the center of Idyllwild leads to Tahquitz Peak, the second-
highest peak in California, and a lookout tower with sweeping views of the Palm
Springs area, the San Jacinto Mountains, and (on a clear day) the Channel Islands.
The total elevation gain is 2,300 feet. This is a favorite trail of several U.S.
Forest Service rangers because the scenic views begin almost immediately. You can
make this hike as short or as long as you want and still get rewarded with views that
you'll remember for years to come. On this trail, all hikers must carry a wilderness
permit; they are available at the Idyllwild Ranger Office. Keep in mind that the views
are greatly obscured on hazy days.*
*OPTION: Make this an overnight hike by continuing another 2 miles to Tahquitz
Valley, where you can set up camp near a year-round stream. An overnight camping
permit is required.*

🚶 Look for the sign for the South Ridge Trail at the north
corner of the parking area. Follow the trail into a dense forest of
pine, spruce, and manzanita. Soon you'll pass a large wooden sign
welcoming you to the San Jacinto Wilderness. The next mile follows
a series of moderate switchbacks uphill past live oaks, manzanita, and
many rocky outcroppings. After approximately 1.5 miles, the trail
levels for about a mile and passes through a wide rocky clearing before
resuming a strenuous uphill course, via switchbacks, to the peak.
Just before the switchbacks begin, you'll come to a wide clearing with
great views of the mountains to the west. This is a good turnaround
point for those looking for a shorter, moderate hike. At mile 2.6,

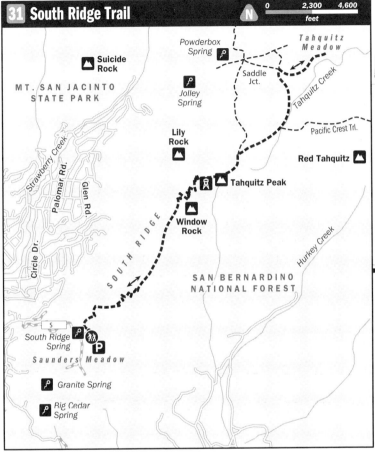

Suicide Rock

MT. SAN JACINTO STATE PARK

Powderbox Spring

Tahquitz Meadow

Saddle Jct.

Jolley Spring

Lily Rock

Tahquitz Creek

Pacific Crest Trl.

Red Tahquitz

Tahquitz Peak

Strawberry Creek

Palomar Rd.

Glen Rd.

Circle Dr.

SOUTH RIDGE

Window Rock

Hurkey Creek

SAN BERNARDINO NATIONAL FOREST

South Ridge Spring

Saunders Meadow

Granite Spring

Big Cedar Spring

you'll come to Window Rock, a striking viewpoint framed by several large boulders. One ranger likes to do this as a sunrise hike, arriving at the trailhead before dawn and hiking up to Window Rock in time to watch the sun come up over the Garner Valley. "You'll never seen another sunrise like it again," he told me.

The next mile is a strenuous climb via switchbacks to Tahquitz Peak. At 3.6 miles, you'll reach a three-way junction; follow the trail to the right to get to Tahquitz Peak; the trail to Saddle Junction, which goes straight, leads to the Pacific Crest Trail and Tahquitz Valley. From the junction, it's a short uphill walk to the base of a fire lookout tower, where you can rest and refuel before heading back. The views from the tower's base are superb, but you can climb the steps to the deck of the lookout for an even better vantage point. The lookout is closed during the winter and early spring, but is staffed by volunteers from May to September.

Those who want to camp overnight should retrace their route to Saddle Junction and turn right (left takes you back to Idyllwild and Tahquitz View Road). Follow the Saddle Junction Trail about 0.5 miles to the Pacific Crest Trail and turn right. After about 0.4 miles make a left; then, at the next trail junction, turn right and follow signs for Tahquitz Valley. The hike from Saddle Junction to Tahquitz Valley is moderate and follows a gradual downhill path.

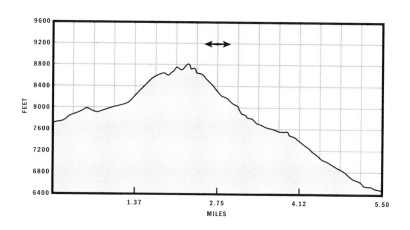

Don't forget to pick up an overnight camping permit at the Idyllwild Ranger Station before heading out.

Beware of rattlesnakes on the trail; they are a common sight during the hot summer and fall months. This is a year-round trail, but keep in mind that can get quite hot in summer and be covered with ice and snow during winter. Check with the Idyllwild Ranger Station, (909) 382-2922, for updates and road conditions.

DIRECTIONS: From Idyllwild, drive south on CA 243 to Saunders Meadow Road (the Idyllwild Café is on the corner). Turn left and follow the road up hill to Pine Avenue. Make a left, then a right on Tahquitz View Drive. Follow the paved road until it ends at a sign for the South Ridge Trail. Turn right and take the unpaved fire road up a steep mile to the trailhead. If you don't have a four-wheel-drive vehicle, park on the street just below the fire road's entrance, being mindful of private property and NO TRESPASSING signs. This will add another strenuous uphill mile to the hike, as well as a steep downhill mile.

GPS Trailhead Coordinates	31 SOUTH RIDGE TO TAHQUITZ PEAK
UTM zone (WGS 84):	11S
Easting:	0528253.7
Northing:	3732677.8
Latitude:	N33° 44.0936'
Longitude:	W116° 41.7680'

32 Spitler Peak Trail

SCENERY: ✿ ✿ ✿ ✿	DISTANCE: *11 miles*
TRAIL CONDITION: ✿ ✿ ✿	HIKING TIME: *4–5 hours*
CHILDREN: *Not recommended*	OUTSTANDING FEATURES: *manzanita,*
DIFFICULTY: ✿ ✿ ✿ ✿	*chaparral, excellent views of Palm Springs and the*
SOLITUDE: ✿ ✿ ✿	*Coachella Valley*

This strenuous single-track trail offers a steady 5-mile ascent past thick chaparral and oak forest to the Pacific Crest Trail and wide-open views of mountains and desert. From the Pacific Crest Trail, it's 0.5 miles to a trail split, where one branch takes you another 0.5 strenuous miles to the top of Spitler Peak. Total elevation gain is 2,600 feet.

OPTION: Make this an overnight hike by turning left at the Pacific Crest Trail junction and walking approximately 1 mile to Apache Springs, a tree-shaded clearing with primitive campsites and a year-round stream. An overnight camping permit is required.

🏃🏃 Look for the brown Spitler Peak Trail sign and begin walking south, then east, on the packed dirt trail. The first 1.5 miles are a gentle climb past thick manzanita, sage, and other desert shrubs. At 2 miles, you'll start to get nice views of Garner Valley and the San Jacinto Mountains to the northwest. The trail continues steadily uphill toward Spitler Peak, moving in and out of dense forest and through wide-open clearings. At about 3.5 miles, the switchbacks get shorter and noticeably steeper, until you reach the saddle at 5 miles, marked by a barely decipherable wooden sign. Stop here and rest while you soak up the stunning views of Palm Springs and the surrounding Coachella Valley. This is a good turnaround point for those looking for a solidly appealing moderate hike with a total 2,000 feet elevation gain. From here, it's another mile (and 600 feet of elevation gain) to Spitler Peak.

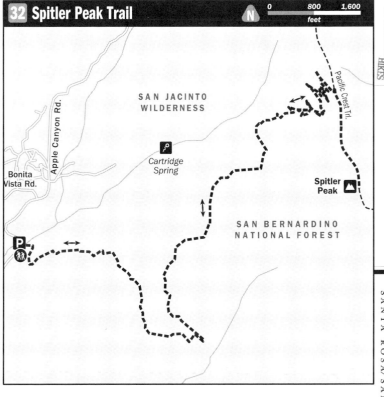

0   800   1,600
feet

SAN JACINTO
WILDERNESS

Apple Canyon Rd.

Pacific Crest Trl.

Cartridge
Spring

Bonita
Vista Rd.

Spitler
Peak

SAN BERNARDINO
NATIONAL FOREST

To continue to Spitler Peak, turn right on the Pacific Crest Trail and walk about 0.5 miles to a trail split marked by a cairn, or small pile of stones. Turn right and follow the narrow trail as it snakes up the mountain for about 0.5 miles to the top, where you'll be treated to a 360-degree view of mountains, desert, and ocean. From here, you can retrace your route to the parking lot or walk north on the Pacific Crest Trail for about a mile to the turnoff for Apache Springs, a good place to set up camp and spend the night.

This is a good hike for solitude; we encountered only two other hikers on a Saturday afternoon in early April. It's best done in early spring or late fall. Gnats rule the area in the summer, and it can get icy around the peak in winter.

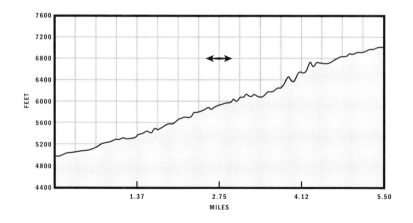

DIRECTIONS: From the Palm Springs area, take CA 111 east to
CA 74, then follow CA 74 south about 33 miles to Apple Canyon
Road. Turn right and go uphill about 3 miles to a sign for the Spitler
Peak Trail. Park in the large lot; a National Forest Adventure or
Golden Eagle pass is required. (See Backcountry Advice for more
information.)

ALTERNATE: From Idyllwild drive 5 miles south on CA 243, then
turn left on SR 74. Go about 4 miles to Apple Canyon Road and
turn left. Go uphill about 3 miles to a sign for the Spitler Peak
Trail. Park in the large lot; a National Forest Adventure or Golden
Eagle pass is required.

GPS Trailhead Coordinates	32 SPITLER PEAK TRAIL
UTM zone (WGS 84):	11S
Easting:	0532312.7
Northing:	3728522.5
Latitude:	N33° 41.8753'
Longitude:	W116° 39.1313'

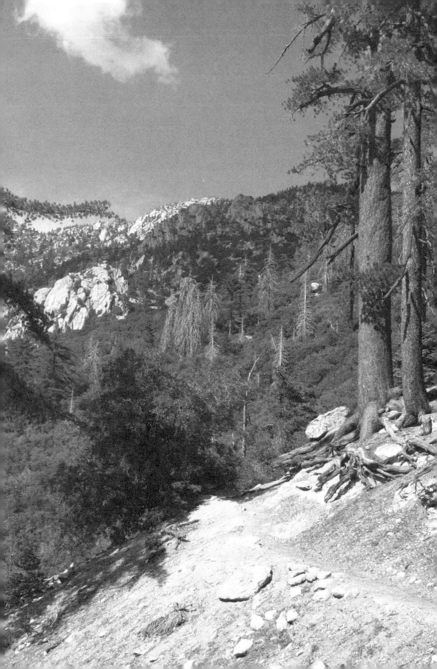

Appendix A: Hikes by Category

Overnight Hikes (continued)

Index

INDEX

OVERNIGHT HIKES

OVERNIGHT HIKES

INDEX

About the Author

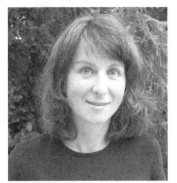

A native of suburban Philadelphia, Laura Randall lived in Washington, D.C. and San Juan, Puerto Rico, before moving to Southern California in 1999. Her byline can be found in a variety of newspapers and consumer magazines, including the *Los Angeles Times, The Washington Post, Sunset, Backpacker,* and *The Christian Science Monitor.* She resides in the San Gabriel Valley and is the author of *60 Hikes within 60 Miles: Los Angeles* (Menasha Ridge Press).

CHECK OUT THESE OTHER GREAT TITLES FROM MENASHA RIDGE PRESS!

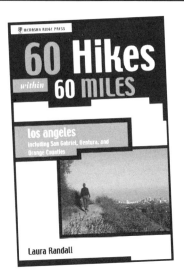

60 HIKES WITHIN 60 MILES: LOS ANGELES

Including San Gabriel, Ventura, and Orange Counties

by Laura Randall
0-89732-638-5 • 978-0-89732-638-4
$16.95
6 x 9, paperback
181 maps, photographs, index

There are fabulous trails throughout the Los Angeles region, and *60 Hikes within 60 Miles: Los Angeles* shows readers how to quickly drive to and enjoy the best hikes from the San Gabriel Mountains to the Pacific Ocean.

The guide is packed with information on hiking in high altitudes, including avoiding high-altitude sickness, steering clear of mountain lions, and what to do in the event of a lightning storm. Two expanded sections in the guide give detailed information on hiking with kids and hiking with dogs.

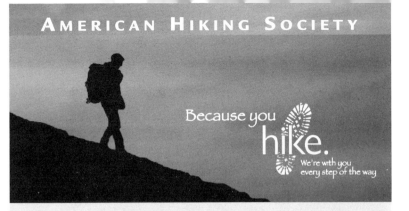

AMERICAN HIKING SOCIETY

Because you **hike.**
We're with you
every step of the way

American Hiking Society gives voice to the more than 75 million Americans who hike and is the only national organization that promotes and protects foot trails, the natural areas that surround them and the hiking experience. Our work is inspiring and challenging, and is built on three pillars:

Policy & Advocacy: We work with Congress and federal agencies to ensure funding for trails, the preservation of natural areas, and the protection of the hiking experience.

Volunteer Programs, Outreach & Education: We organize and coordinate nationally recognized programs - including Volunteer Vacations and National Trails Day® - that help keep our trails open, safe, and enjoyable.

Trail Grants & Assistance: We support trail clubs and hiking organizations by providing technical assistance, resources, and grant funding so that trails and trail corridors across the country are maintained and preserved.

You can help and support these efforts. Become an American Hiking Society volunteer and member today!

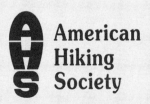

American Hiking Society

1422 Fenwick Lane · Silver Spring, MD 20910 · (301) 565-6704
www.AmericanHiking.org · info@AmericanHiking.org

DEAR CUSTOMERS AND FRIENDS,

SUPPORTING YOUR INTEREST IN OUTDOOR ADVENTURE, travel, and an active lifestyle is central to our operations, from the authors we choose to the locations we detail to the way we design our books. Menasha Ridge Press was incorporated in 1982 by a group of veteran outdoorsmen and professional outfitters. For 25 years now, we've specialized in creating books that benefit the outdoors enthusiast.

Almost immediately, Menasha Ridge Press earned a reputation for revolutionizing outdoors- and travel-guidebook publishing. For such activities as canoeing, kayaking, hiking, backpacking, and mountain biking, we established new standards of quality that transformed the whole genre, resulting in outdoor-recreation guides of great sophistication and solid content. Menasha Ridge continues to be outdoor publishing's greatest innovator.

The folks at Menasha Ridge Press are as at home on a white-water river or mountain trail as they are editing a manuscript. The books we build for you are the best they can be, because we're responding to your needs. Plus, we use and depend on them ourselves.

We look forward to seeing you on the river or the trail. If you'd like to contact us directly, join in at www.trekalong.com or visit us at www.menasharidge.com. We thank you for your interest in our books and the natural world around us all.

SAFE TRAVELS,

Bob Sehlinger

BOB SEHLINGER
PUBLISHER